get the med

medium books to

find out how to really

heal ♡

THE INTEGRATIVE NUTRITION

Cookbook

Simple Recipes for Health and Happiness

Joshua Rosenthal

FOUNDER AND DIRECTOR, INSTITUTE FOR INTEGRATIVE NUTRITION

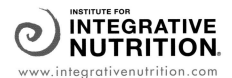

INSTITUTE FOR
INTEGRATIVE NUTRITION®

www.integrativenutrition.com

The Integrative Nutrition Cookbook: Simple Recipes for Health and Happiness

ISBN: 978-1-941908-12-9 (hardcover)
ISBN: 978-1-941908-13-6 (e-book)

Copyright © 2018 by Integrative Nutrition, Inc.

Library of Congress Control Number: 2018938539

Published by Integrative Nutrition, Inc., New York, NY
www.integrativenutrition.com

Notice: This book is not intended to replace recommendations or advice from physicians or other healthcare providers. Rather, it is intended to help you make informed decisions about your health and to cooperate with your healthcare provider in a joint quest for optimal wellness. If you suspect you have a medical problem, we urge you to seek medical attention from a competent healthcare provider.

Printed in China

10 9 8 7 6 5 4 3 2 1

First Edition

Special thanks to Michaela Rowland and Lula Brown for their support and dedication to the success of this project. Additional thanks to Tim Tate, Angela Singer, Joline Seavey, and Erika Ramirez.

OTHER TITLES BY JOSHUA ROSENTHAL

TABLE OF CONTENTS

FOREWORD

As a child, I remember elders in my community talking about their health challenges and how doctors assured them that food had little or no effect on disease. With advances in every field of health and nutritional science, it's now widely known that a wholesome diet and a vibrant lifestyle are key for a long and robust life.

Despite this information, the vast majority of people today struggle to eat well for a variety of reasons, including not having the skill and time to prepare healthy food. By providing simple, tasty, and nourishing recipes, *The Integrative Nutrition Cookbook* solves that problem. In this much-needed food preparation guide, Joshua Rosenthal does what he does best: With efficiency and simplicity, he opens you to the full spectrum of culinary experience, from vegan to omnivore, while encouraging quality choices that mirror your current lifestyle and state of emotional and physical health.

Like Joshua, I enjoy nothing more than stepping into my kitchen to cook, so I'm thrilled that he's put together these recipes for you. As one of the most innovative teachers in nutrition today, Joshua is pioneering new thinking that excludes no one. People with an interest in improving their lives can find exceptional value in the dietary teachings he provides in his programs. And these teachings, including the recipes in this book, represent the most effective nutrition and food therapies available.

In the modern world, emotions are a guiding force for nearly everyone. More than anyone I've observed, Joshua understands the nature and value of emotional clarity and how to guide his students with simple, coherent steps that result in optimal nutrition.

Now I want to emphasize a few topics that complement this essential cookbook.

The first step to good health is an open mind and heart. When you engage in calming practices like simple, silent contemplation, meditation, prayer, or mantra, you set the stage for optimal health. When your mind is calm and clear, you discover that most challenges in life actually have an inner function that sparks your curiosity to explore what's going on for you.

As you begin to incorporate these focusing practices, you tend to naturally make better nutritional choices. There are few better teachers than Joshua Rosenthal to guide you through basic cooking to nourish your body on all levels. With a little practice, preparing simple, flavorful food can become not only enjoyable, but a virtually effortless process.

Simpler cooking is better, as complicated recipes can be harder to digest and often contain more irritants and even toxic ingredients. So let's stick with the basics as I introduce you to Joshua's collection of nutrient-dense, delicious recipes.

Dozens of factors play a role in vibrant health and mental clarity, simple and clean food being one of them. Other fundamental factors that set the stage for health are clean air, sunlight, and pure water. Inhaling fresh air and getting adequate sunlight, even when there's cloud coverage, supports vitality in all bodily systems, including the bones, tissues and fluids. Sunlight also has been used traditionally, as well as in modern medicine, to brighten the mind and boost the spirit.

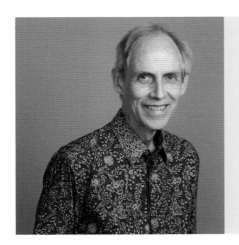

"Like Joshua, I enjoy nothing more than stepping into my kitchen to cook, so I'm thrilled that he's put together these recipes for you."

Air is often overlooked as a nutrient, but it's actually crucial to good health. Are you breathing enough clean air? When you go from the city to the country, for example, you notice the change in air quality immediately, and you feel energized. When you're breathing toxic air, your immune system is compromised and you're more likely to get sick, have congested skin, and suffer digestive issues. When you breathe vibrant air and get exposure to sunlight, you become activated and feel light and focused.

Then we have water—you've probably heard many times how key it is for health. Male adults are 60% water and females about 55%. Given that statistic, you can imagine how crucial it is to keep your body hydrated. When your system is lubricated with fresh water, your digestion, circulation, and all other functions run smoothly. Water also helps regulate appetite. Often when you're hungry, you just need a glass of water, a cup of herbal tea, vegetable juice, a piece of melon, coconut water, or another high-quality beverage. When you're hydrated, your hunger calibrates so you only crave food when your body truly needs it.

The benefits of water are numerous, but all you really need to know is that you should quench your thirst with pure water by itself and as an ingredient in foods such as soups and healthy drinks, every day.

So it's clear: Even before learning about food preparation, the key nutrients to consume are clean sources of water and air, along with daily exposure to sunlight. Of course, avoid overexposure and sunburn.

After you've given your body these foundational nutrients, consider that your food fuels the building blocks for every part of your body. When making nutritional choices, choose the highest quality food available, because food is much more than just fuel; it also contributes to cell renewal and longevity. When you fill your body with toxic, processed food, you compromise your health and make yourself far more susceptible to chronic illness. When you consume organic fruits and vegetables, healthy sources of protein and fats, and unrefined complex carbohydrates, you can reach optimal health.

By experimenting with Joshua's recipes, you'll be able to replace processed ingredients in your diet with nutritious ones. You'll find great ideas for appetizers, entrees, and side dishes, as well as healthy beverages; even desserts are an available option. These recipes are the perfect place to start when creating a balanced relationship with food and cooking. Cooking and eating well is one of the surest ways to create a strong, vital body and mind.

Paul Pitchford
author of Healing with Whole Foods:
Asian Traditions and Modern Nutrition

OUR MISSION

Integrative Nutrition is not just a school—it's a movement. Our mission is to play a crucial role in improving health and happiness, and through that process, create a ripple effect that transforms the world. The ripple effect happens when one person learns how to truly heal their bodies by themselves through food and lifestyle, and then inspire someone else to do the same, and so on. If each person affects 10 people, that will eventually amount to tens of thousands of people and even millions over time. That's the ripple effect in action.

A big part of spreading the ripple effect is teaching people how to get comfortable in the kitchen. The truth is that the body knows how to heal itself by itself, and if you focus on eating food for your bio-individual type and drinking enough water, most imbalances will improve naturally.

Early on, one of my teachers, Michio Kushi, told me that cooking is really a spiritual practice. While in the kitchen, you prepare nourishment for yourself, which is crucial to your health and happiness. And when you extend that nourishment to others by preparing meals for your friends and family, you create connection and show love. I always say a simple meal made with love is better than any fancy meal eaten in a restaurant. This is why it's important to take a moment before you step into the kitchen to center your energy since your energy goes directly into the food you make.

My Mom's Cholent Recipe

Cholent is a traditional stew. It's simmered overnight and eaten the next day. The main ingredients are beans and potatoes. Sometimes meat is added. This dish is very grounding and perfect for the colder months. My dear mother would make it on special occasions, and it would help me feel warm and grounded.

Spiritual communities often choose the healthiest, happiest person to do the cooking because they want their food filled with positive energy. This impacts the whole community—the chef plays a critically important role. When the whole community is eating beautiful food filled with love and positivity, harmony is strengthened.

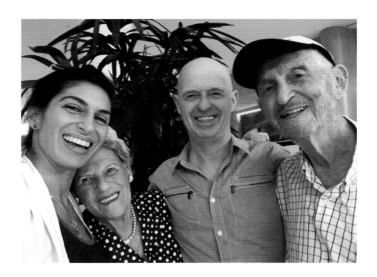

Cholent

Prep time: 15 minutes
Cook time: 12 hours

Ingredients
Serves 6–8

4 potatoes
½ cup barley
1 cup small beans
2 large onions
1 tsp paprika
3 tbsps extra virgin
   olive oil
Salt, to taste
Black pepper, to taste

Method

• Wash beans, barley, and potatoes.

• Cut onions and potatoes into large chunks.

• Place all the above into a heavy pot.

• Add remaining ingredients.

• Add water to cover ingredients, plus
  2 inches more.

• Cover and cook 12 hours.

• Lift cover and check from time to time.

• Add salt an hour before servings.

Optional ingredients:

Add one winter squash.

My mother would also add beef bones to this dish. We would eat the bone marrow as a special treat!

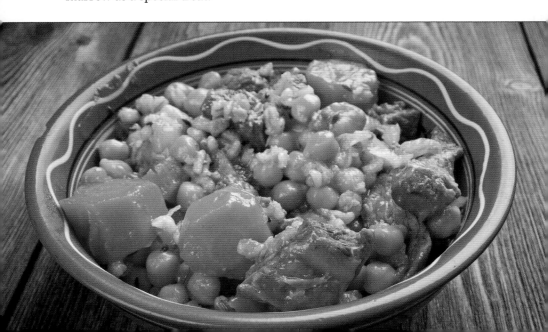

If you're feeling negative, whether you've gotten into a fight with your partner or had a bad day at work, it's not a good time to be cooking or eating. That energy will go into the food and may foster negativity in yourself and anyone you're feeding.

To clear your energy before cooking, try this exercise: Drop your chin to your chest, breathe in through your nose and out through your mouth. Allow your stomach to expand completely while inhaling. Then, contract while exhaling. Clear your mind by telling yourself that you have nowhere to go and nothing to do except be in this moment. Center yourself. Once you're feeling clear, light a candle to help make this a special moment.

Cooking is sacred, and it's an art. In fact, it's the only art that actually enters our body and creates our future. Long after the flavor in your mouth is gone, the food you eat is digested in your belly and helps create your cells, tissues, hair, skin, thoughts, and even your feelings, so this is a very important process. If you make the experience special, your food will be special. People will feel the love in your food. Try it!

It's not practical to be totally perfect with your food all the time; just choose the healthiest option 90% of the time and eat whatever you want the other 10%. That's my foolproof method for sustainable health and vibrant energy—I call it the 90/10 diet. If you put too much pressure on yourself to be perfectly perfect, you're going to run into problems. Just know that the faster the food is made, the faster it's eaten and the less nourishing and satisfying it is. You're saving time but losing energy.

With this book, I'd like to encourage you to take a step back and make every meal an event. They don't have to be fancy, but your digestion, weight, and mindset will improve if you slow down and make time to chew your food.

This book is for everyone—vegans, vegetarians, omnivores, and carnivores. I've put a lot of thought and care into creating recipes that will be easy to prepare and also nurturing for your body and soul. As you begin experimenting with these recipes, let me know how it goes. Share comments and photos by tagging @nutritionschool on Twitter and Instagram. I can't wait to see your beautiful photos. Please spread the ripple effect by sharing these recipes with family, friends, and clients.

WHY I WROTE THIS

C ooking is often overcomplicated, and my intention in writing this book is to teach you that it can be very simple. On TV, food is glamorized so much that viewers become intimidated and reluctant to try the recipes. I've done the opposite and put together very basic recipes that you'll actually want to make and eat. When you start being able to create food that tastes really good and makes your body feel vibrant, you're going to become more comfortable in the kitchen. Soon enough, you'll be creating exciting new concoctions of your own that you'll want to share with others.

For now, step away from exotic ingredients and fancy cutting methods. Trust me—homemade food is a precious gift, and you have all the skills to start right now! A big ingredient missing in modern nutrition is what I like to call Vitamin L, for *love*. This is a major reason the food you make at home is so different from the food you eat at a restaurant. So often at restaurants, everything is fine and friendly in the dining room and you have a great experience, but the truth is that the chefs in the kitchen are often stressed and sometimes underpaid, leading them to care very little about putting love into the food they're making, even if cooking is their passion. For this reason, it's important to try to make most of your food at home. As you start cooking more, notice how you feel after eating a meal you or a loved one prepared at home versus how you feel after a restaurant meal. It may be the exact same food, but I bet you'll get that "something's missing" feeling. You guessed it— Vitamin L.

I wrote this book to support you in putting love into the food you make so that you can share that love with your clients, family, friends, and most importantly, yourself. I've included foods that cater to many different dietary restrictions. I've gone through a lot of experimentation with my own approach to food, and I've seen thousands of people have life-changing epiphanies in this area. No one diet works for everyone.

Dairy will work for some people but not others. Some will want to eat meat and others will want to be vegan. I have also seen a lot of differences between the types of food men like to eat and the types of food women like to eat. Bio-individuality is the core principle here—one person's food is another person's poison, and no two people will thrive on the exact same diet. I created this cookbook to be a universal tool that everyone will find helpful, no matter what your dietary preferences are.

Even if you have no dietary restrictions and just love good food, you're going to find a lot of value in these recipes. Food is transformative, and you'll become so much more connected with your family and friends when you come together to share food. I want to inspire you to get comfortable in the kitchen and start feeding your soul today.

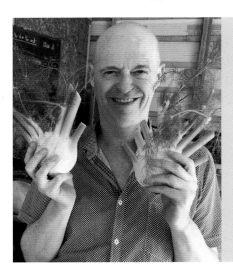

"Homemade food is a precious gift, and you have all the skills to start right now!"

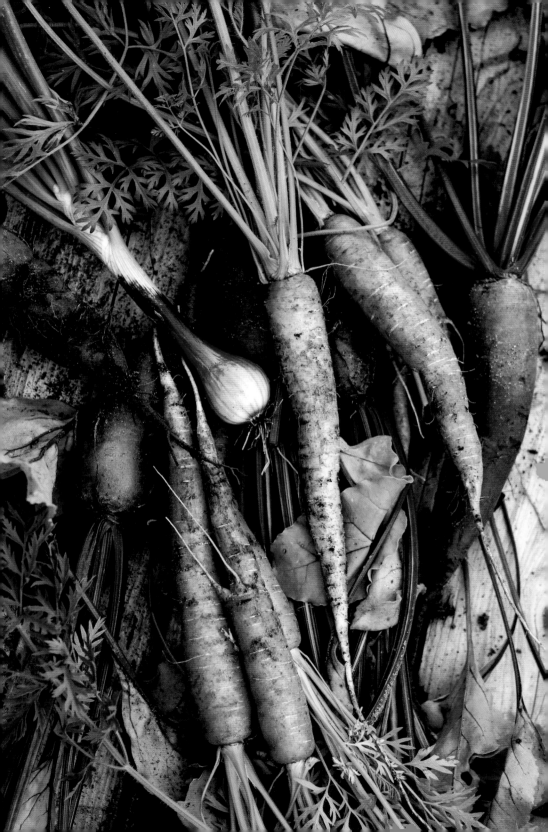

ORGANIC AND LOCAL FOOD

Next, I want to talk about organic and local food. Conventional food is sprayed with chemicals and pesticides, and organic food is grown naturally with no chemicals. The government argues that the nutritional content of conventional and organic food is the same, but many experts strongly disagree.

Organics is one of the fastest-growing categories in the food industry, despite the fact that it costs more than conventional. The goal in many countries has always been to make the price of food as low as possible so that as many people as possible can buy it. The organic movement started when a subset of people realized that a certain demographic cares a lot about the quality of their food and will pay more for it so they can avoid getting sick and having to pay high doctor's bills down the road. Global organic sales are currently well over $63 billion[1] and are expected to exceed $100 billion[2] this year.

The bottom line is that we should all try to eat organic as much as possible, but it's more important to simply focus on whole foods like vegetables, fruits, and whole grains. Yes, organic is healthier, but conventional broccoli is better than no broccoli at all.

---

1 Global organic sales reach $63 billion, U.S. is largest market. http://www.agprofessional .com/news/Global-organic-sales-reach-63-billion-US-is-largest-market--212753341.html.

2 Global organic food and beverages market to reach $104 billion. http://www .ecologyandfarming.com/global-organic-food-beverages-market-reach-104-billion/.

Today, organic food can be coming to you from China, Brazil, or anywhere in the world where it's available. Given the environmental crisis, this is making a lot of people wonder whether importing organic food far distances is actually worth it. That's where local food comes in—many people believe that local is more important than organic since when you eat locally, the food will be seasonal by default and support your body in your environment.

I don't think that most people realize how far their food travels to get to them and all the resources transportation involves. All this travel causes food to lose its freshness, and it's a waste of fuel.

It's an ongoing process to make intelligent choices for yourself from day to day. For example, New York grows more apples than New York consumes, and yet, you can go to the store and the apples for sale are from Washington State.

Often, we try to do everything at once—go vegetarian, give up coffee, and ban sugar, and we end up overwhelmed. Start by simply eating more fruits and vegetables, ideally organic, but not necessarily all of the time. Take baby steps if necessary—buy canned vegetables and frozen vegetables, even if they're not organic, and aim to get that food into your system; that's a great place to start. Then, later, once you get used to this new style of eating, you can start to expand your knowledge and prioritize organic food in your life.

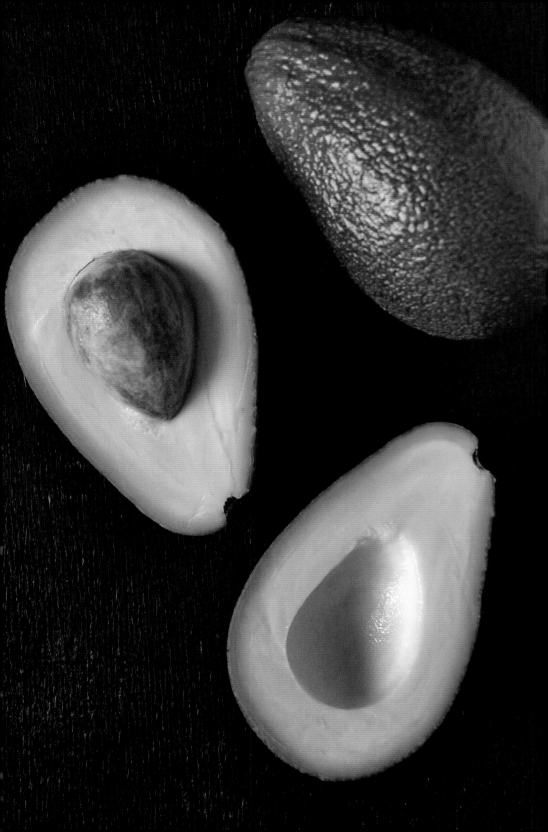

THE DIRTY DOZEN AND THE CLEAN FIFTEEN

The big thing about organic is it avoids synthetic pesticides and doesn't put chemicals into the groundwater. Organic produce also doesn't affect wildlife, reduces fossil fuel consumption, and tastes better. A lot of fruits and vegetables have pesticide residue that doesn't always come off with basic washing. For some people, it's challenging to have access to organic food for financial and regional reasons. The Dirty Dozen™ and The Clean Fifteen™ are helpful tools when deciding which foods to buy organic.

The Dirty Dozen includes foods where pesticides are sprayed directly onto the part that we eat, which makes them more hazardous, especially for children. There are also a few additional items that fall under The Dirty Dozen + list—and it's best to buy those organic whenever possible—but the primary 12 are most important to buy organic. These lists cover only fruits and vegetables, but it's important to remember that animal food should also be high quality and humane. I think that the fear and trauma the animal goes through translates to the food and then to the human, so it's important to buy only local, sustainable, organic meat.

The Clean Fifteen is made up of foods that have an outer covering, so when they're sprayed you're not exposed to the chemicals since you're only eating the inside. Or, for other fruits and vegetables, they're deemed clean simply because producers don't use a lot of pesticides on them, if any. The vegetable with the lowest level of pesticides is an onion. It's so cool that it has this special wrapping and the pesticides can't get in there.

Ninety percent of Americans are unaware of what goes into their body and their children's bodies every day. Celebrities and pop culture seem more important these days, but they're really just distractions from what creates a healthy planet and healthy future. Don't fall into this trap.

Check out The Dirty Dozen and The Clean Fifteen here. Write them down or print them out to use whenever you go grocery shopping. Keep in mind that these two lists are constantly being updated to reflect the latest findings and agricultural changes, so please find the most recent versions from a reputable Internet source such as the Environmental Working Group (EWG) website noted below.

Each year analysts at the Environmental Working Group (EWG) create lists of fruits and vegetables that have been found to have the most and least amounts of pesticide residue. Their work is based on laboratory tests done by the USDA Pesticide Testing Program and the Food and Drug Administration. EWG is a not-for-profit environmental research organization dedicated to improving public health and protecting the environment. In general, more delicate foods, such as leafy greens and fruits with soft peels like apples and peaches, tend to have higher amounts of residue. Heartier foods, like avocadoes, pineapples, and onions, tend to have less. Use these lists to help you make food choices, and if you can't buy all organic, consider these lists to help you prioritize what to buy organic. Check out their website at **www.ewg.org/foodnews.**

The Dirty Dozen+

1. Strawberries
2. Spinach
3. Nectarines
4. Apples
5. Peaches
6. Pears
7. Cherries
8. Grapes
9. Celery
10. Tomatoes
11. Sweet bell peppers
12. Potatoes
13. Hot peppers +

+ Dirty Dozen PLUS

The Clean Fifteen

1. Sweet Corn*
2. Avocadoes
3. Pineapples
4. Cabbage
5. Onions
6. Frozen sweet peas
7. Papayas*
8. Asparagus
9. Mangoes
10. Eggplant
11. Honeydew Melon
12. Kiwi
13. Cantaloupe
14. Cauliflower
15. Grapefruit

*A small amount of sweet corn, papaya, and summer squash sold in the United States is produced from genetically modified seeds. Buy organic varieties of these crops if you want to avoid genetically modified produce.

SEASONAL GUIDE

In many parts of the world, winter, spring, summer, and fall have relatively different temperatures. This calls for different foods since differences in weather give us different crops. Mother Nature gives us what we need to be our healthiest selves during each season. For example, we get squash and potatoes in the fall to help our bodies warm up as we enter colder weather and sprouts in the spring to cleanse ourselves after winter.

Summer provides lots of fresh, high-water-content fruits and vegetables to hydrate our bodies and replace lost fluids when we're faced with high temperatures that cause us to sweat a lot.

Now I'm going to give you an overview of each season. Keep in mind, depending on where you live, your seasonal foods will vary. Use a sustainable online source to see what's in season for you at any time.

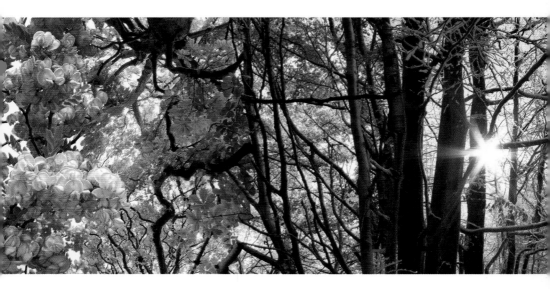

Spring

New beginnings
Cleaning out the home
Cleansing the body and mind
Leafy greens and sprouts
Fruit and vegetable juices

Suggestions:

Citrus
Avocado
Asparagus
Zucchini
Seafood

Summer

Laughter and fun
Vigorous exercise
Sweating
Raw fruits and vegetables
Hydrating liquids and foods

Suggestions:

Celery
Berries
Watermelon
Tomatoes
Snap peas

Fall

Productivity
Communication
Rest
Yoga and qigong
Less fruit

Suggestions:

Pumpkin
Nuts
Mushrooms
Kale
Cabbage

Winter

Introspection
Time with loved ones
Rest
Minimal fruits
More cooked foods than raw foods

Suggestions:

Protein and carbohydrates
Deep sea fish
Seaweed
Chestnuts
Miso

PANTRY BASICS

C ooking is a primary component of health, and it starts with having basic ingredients on hand at all times—make it easy for yourself! Having a well-stocked kitchen will encourage you to cook more and experiment with different flavors so you can discover what types of food you really enjoy and eat homemade food filled with love regularly. When you do this, you'll start to notice profound changes in your body and mind.

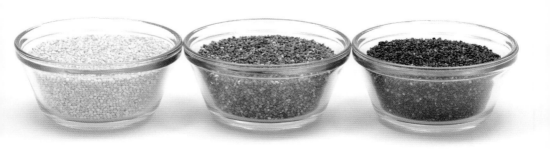

I'm going to outline some kitchen staples for you. Don't feel pressured to have everything on this list. Keep in mind that condiments and spices will change depending on your personal tastes; stock up on the ones you love and find replacements for the ones you don't.

Nuts and seeds also have a long shelf life. Stock up on these so you can add healthy fat, fiber, and protein to any meal very quickly.

While you'll typically buy produce based on what you're making on a given day, there are a few staples that keep for two weeks or longer in the refrigerator or pantry and are convenient to have on hand.

Grains, beans, and legumes are easy to keep in your pantry because they have a very long shelf life. If the conditions are good, these items will last in tightly sealed jars for years. For this reason, buying grains, beans, and legumes in bulk is a great idea, and it ensures you'll always have some staples around to make a healthy meal when you're feeling hungry and don't have a lot of time.

These are the basics to have in your pantry at all times, which will help you create healthy, delicious meals when you don't have much time. Having healthy basics and condiments readily available will encourage you to get into the kitchen.

Staples

- Vegetable stock
- Tomato sauce
- Canned coconut milk (look for BPA-free)
- Ketchup
- Mustard
- Breadcrumbs (gluten-free or not)
- Nutritional yeast
- Sauerkraut
- Pickles
- Dulse flakes
- Nori sheets
- Organic coffee beans
- Raisins
- Coconut flakes

Healthy Fats

- Extra virgin olive oil
- Coconut oil
- Sesame oil
- Butter or ghee, if tolerated

Vinegars

- Apple cider vinegar
- Balsamic vinegar
- Umeboshi vinegar
- Brown rice vinegar

Spices and Seasonings

- Sea salt
- Himalayan salt
- Herbamare
- Gomasio
- Black pepper
- White pepper
- Bay leaves
- Basil
- Oregano
- Thyme
- Rosemary
- Coriander
- Cumin
- Paprika
- Red pepper flakes
- Cayenne pepper
- Chili powder
- Curry powder
- Turmeric
- Ginger powder
- Onion powder
- Garlic powder
- Cinnamon
- Cacao powder
- Vanilla extract
- Tamari
- Hot sauce

Sweeteners

- Raw honey
- Maple syrup
- Coconut palm sugar
- Brown rice syrup
- Dates
- Stevia

Grains

- Kasha
- Millet
- Quinoa
- Rolled oats
- Short grain brown rice
- Whole wheat flour

Beans

- Black beans
- Chickpeas
- Pinto beans
- White beans

Nuts, Nut Butters, and Seeds

- Almonds
- Cashews
- Walnuts
- Pistachios
- Brazil nuts
- Pine nuts
- Almond butter
- Peanut butter
- Pumpkin seeds
- Sunflower seeds
- Sesame seeds
- Flax seeds
- Chia seeds
- Hemp seeds

Produce

- Garlic
- Ginger
- Lemons
- Onions

HOW TO USE THIS COOKBOOK

C ooking nourishes your body and mind on many levels. It slows you down and brings you into the present moment, giving you a chance to nourish yourself and the people you love. By cooking at home, you can control what goes into your body and go back to a simpler way of eating that will be much healthier than anything you get outside the home.

The recipes in this cookbook have been carefully selected to cover all dietary needs in a healthy and accessible way. These recipes seldom include more than 5–7 ingredients, and we encourage readers to repurpose the ingredients they buy for more than one recipe.

I've done some cool things to make it easy for you to navigate this book:

- *Are you looking for a recipe for a specific meal?* Reference the **Table of Contents**. The recipes are divided into sections like **The Main Event** and then into chapters like **Perfect Proteins**.

- *Wondering what you should do with your extra kale?* I included *IIN*sider **Tips** for repurposing your ingredients for other recipes within this cookbook.

- *Aren't familiar with the nutritional information or health benefits of a food?* Check the **Glossary** at the end of the book.

- *Do you have food allergies/intolerances?* If you have food allergies or are interested in making a meal within certain dietary guidelines, there is a section called **Freedom Favorites** with chapters that cover vegan, gluten-free, and vegetarian recipes, to mention a few. Also, all of my recipes have dietary icons right underneath the title. Pretty cool, right?

V Vegan

VG Vegetarian

GF Gluten-Free

DF Dairy-Free

- *There's no community like the IIN community.* Some of my awesome graduates contributed great recipes, and I'm so excited to share them with you. Look out for **Grad Features** in each section.

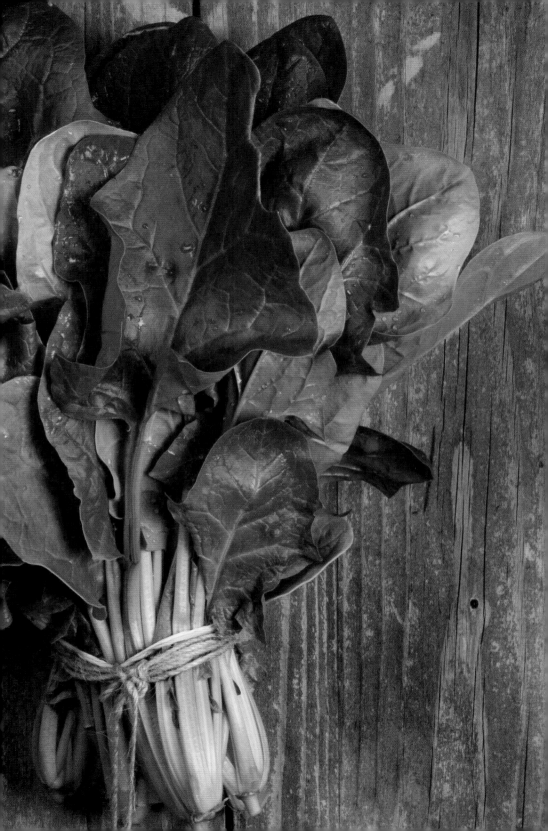

The Main Event

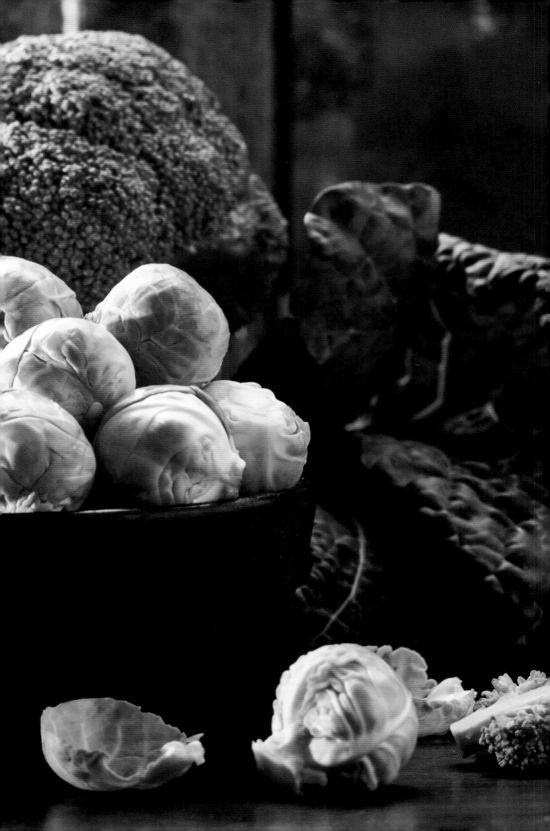

Chapter 1: Delicious Dark Greens

We could all use an extra dose of green vegetables—roasted, steamed, raw, or sautéed—in our diet. Why? Because vegetables, especially dark leafy vegetables, are nutritional powerhouses packed with fiber, calcium, antioxidants and almost every vitamin from A to K. I could write a book on the health benefits of vegetables alone, but for now a few include improved blood circulation, lower cholesterol, healthier intestinal flora, increased energy, improved kidney and liver function, and even clearer congestion. Vegetables can sometimes be challenging to integrate, especially if you usually find them unappetizing. In this chapter, I'll show you how to make green vegetables tasty by pairing them with the perfect, complementary ingredients.

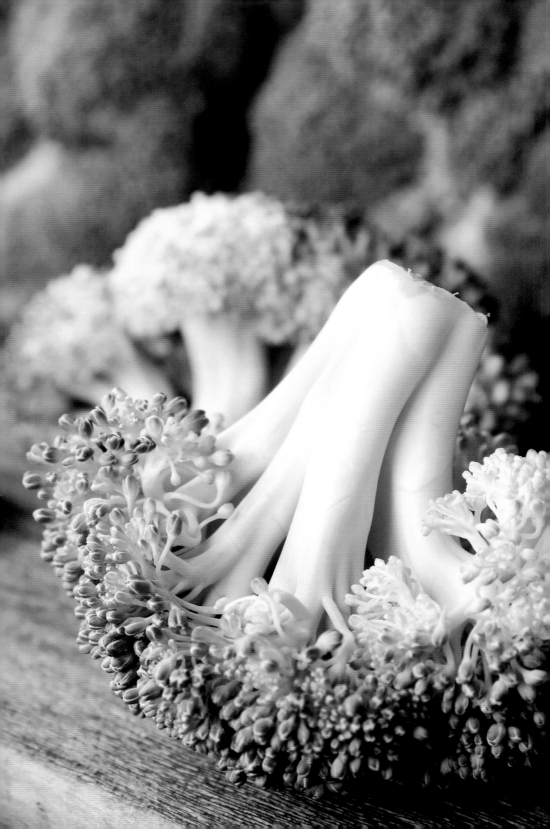

Broccoli and Tempeh Curry with Caramelized Onions Ⓥ ⒼⒻ

Prep time: 15 minutes
Cook time: 35 minutes

Ingredients
Serves 2

3 cups broccoli

1 block tempeh

1 medium yellow onion

3 garlic cloves, minced

1 cup coconut milk

2 tsps curry powder, or to taste

2 tbsps coconut oil

2 tbsps tamari, or to taste

½ cup brown rice or quinoa (optional)

Method

• Bring 4 cups water to a boil.

• Cut broccoli into florets and parboil for 3–4 minutes, or to desired texture. Strain and set aside.

• Bring 2 cups water to a boil. Cut block of tempeh in half the short way, then the long way.

• Parboil tempeh for 5–7 minutes, or until tender. Strain and set aside. Allow to cool, then slice into thin strips.

• Chop onion and garlic.

• Add two tablespoons coconut oil to pan and bring to medium heat.

• Add onions and garlic to pan and cook for 5–7 minutes, or until translucent.

• Add broccoli and tempeh to pan, along with curry powder and tamari.

• Sauté for 5–7 minutes, combining well.

• Add coconut milk, reduce to low heat and cover. Simmer 8–10 minutes.

• Serve as-is or over brown rice or quinoa.

IINsider Tip: If you bought extra tempeh, make the Grilled Tempeh Collard "Tacos" Ⓥ ⒼⒻ *the same week as these, so you can use your tempeh twice. (See page 131.)*

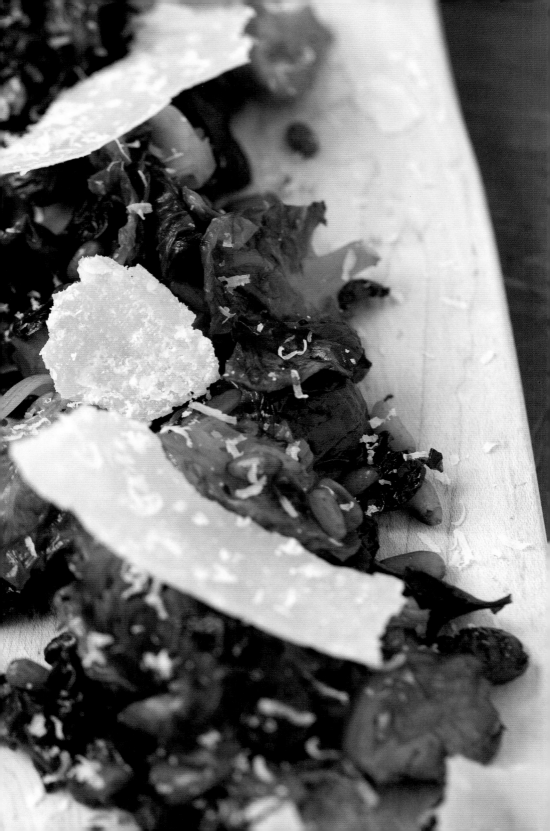

Roasted Brussels Sprouts with Pine Nuts and Dried Cherries (VG) (GF)

Prep time: 15 minutes
Cook time: 30 minutes

Ingredients
Serves 2

2 cups Brussels sprouts

¼ cup dried cherries

¼ cup pine nuts

2 tbsps olive oil

Sea salt, to taste

¼ cup grated
Parmesan cheese
(optional)

Method

• Preheat oven to 350°F.

• Bring 3 cups water to a boil.

• Trim ends and wash Brussels sprouts well.

• Parboil for 7–9 minutes or until fork tender.

• Transfer to large mixing bowl.

• Chop dried cherries into small pieces.

• Toss Brussels sprouts with olive oil, dried cherries, pine nuts, and salt.

• Transfer to baking sheet, ensuring the Brussels sprouts are in one layer, and roast for 15 minutes, or until golden brown.

• Sprinkle with Parmesan if desired and serve.

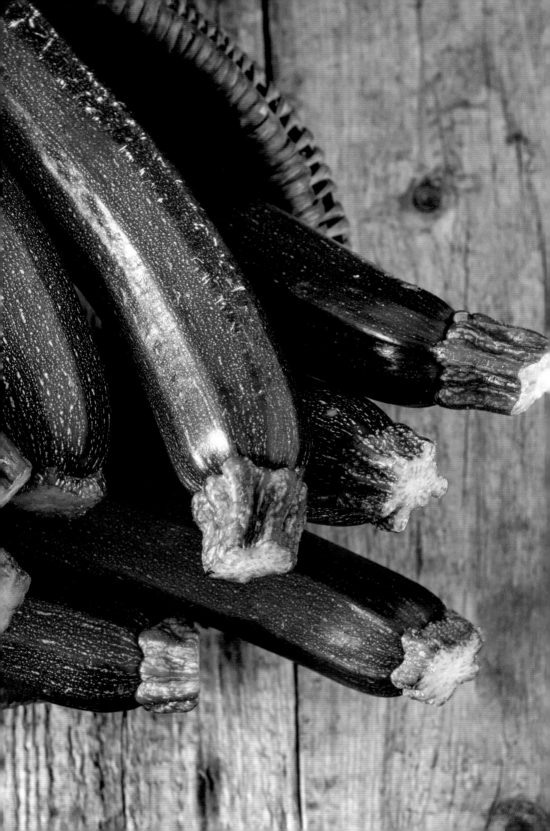

Vegetable and Tofu Stir-Fry

Prep time: 15 minutes
Cook time: 30 minutes

Ingredients
Serves 2

1 medium onion

1 red pepper

1 medium zucchini

1 lb shiitake
mushrooms

1 block tofu

2 tbsps sesame oil

1 tbsp minced ginger

½ cup coconut milk

2 tbsps tamari, or to
taste

1 tbsp honey (optional)

½ cup basmati rice
(optional)

Method

• Wrap raw tofu in paper towels or clean
dishcloth and press with book or other heavy
object for an hour or more to remove as much
liquid as possible.

• Slice onion thin.

• Wash and pat dry pepper and zucchini
and dice.

• Slice mushrooms thin.

• Simmer sesame oil on medium heat in pan
and add onions first. Cook 5–7 minutes or
until translucent.

• Add peppers, zucchini, and mushrooms and
cook for 5–7 minutes until caramelized.

• Slice tofu thin and add to pan. Cook for 5
minutes.

• Add minced ginger, honey, coconut milk, and
tamari.

• Stir well, reduce heat, cover, and simmer for
5 minutes.

• Serve over basmati rice or as-is.

IINsider Tip: Buy extra tofu? Make Dianne Wenz's Pad Thai Salad   *the
same week. (See page 125.)*

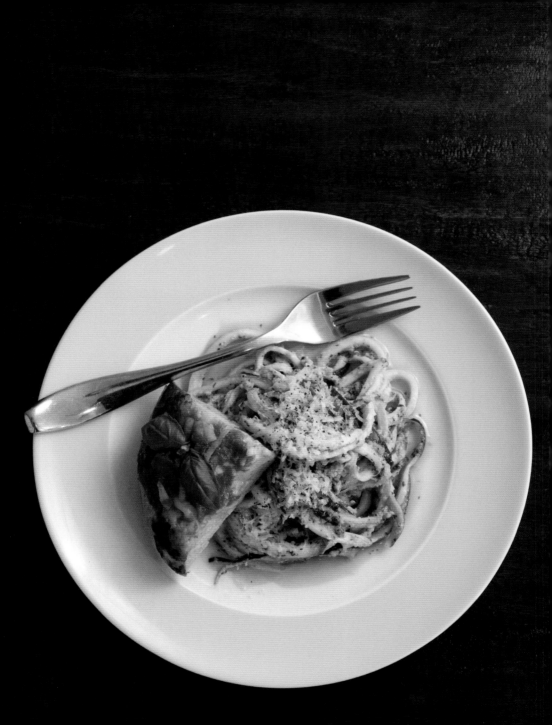

Zucchini Noodles with Pesto and Grilled Focaccia (V)

Prep time: 10 minutes
Cook time: 15 minutes

Ingredients
Serves 2

3 large zucchinis

8 oz focaccia, or two slices

2 bunches basil

½ cup pine nuts, toasted

Juice of 1 lemon

¼ cup extra virgin olive oil

1 tbsp sea salt, to taste

Black pepper, to taste

¼ cup Parmesan cheese (optional)

Method

• Wash, pat dry, and trim zucchini ends. Create noodles using a spiralizer tool.

• Option: Sauté your "noodles" in olive oil over medium-high heat for 4–6 minutes. Add salt and black pepper to taste.

• Wash and dry basil and add to blender with pine nuts, lemon, extra virgin olive oil, and salt.

• Blend until smooth, adding more olive oil and/or water as needed.

• Toss zucchini noodles with pesto and top with Parmesan, if desired.

• Bring 1 tablespoon olive oil to medium heat in pan and toast focaccia in olive oil. Serve alongside pesto-zucchini noodles.

IINsider Tip: Extra zucchini? Make Cauliflower Rice with Grilled Shrimp and Spicy Drizzle (V) (GF) this week and use your zucchini twice. (See page 141.)

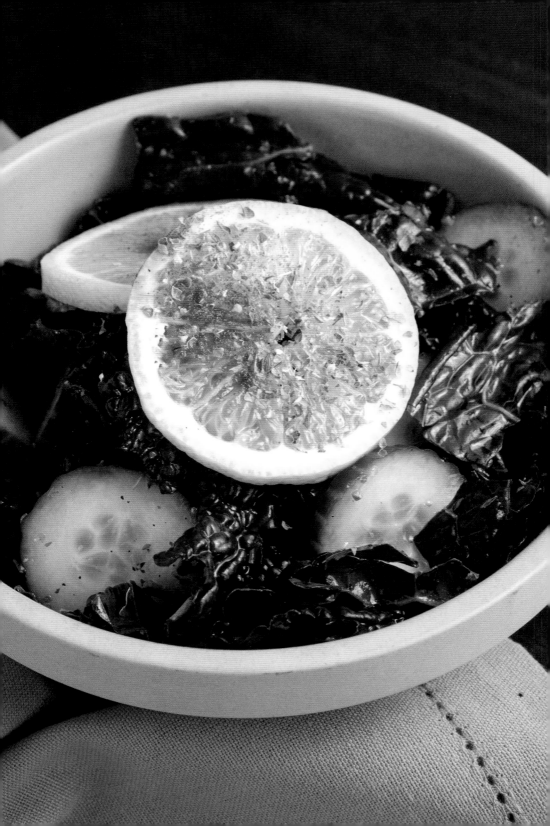

Massaged Kale Salad with Lemon Vinaigrette (V) (GF)

Prep time: 15 minutes
Cook time: 0 minutes

Ingredients
Serves 2

1 large head kale

1 English cucumber

Juice of 2 lemons

3 tbsps extra virgin olive oil

1 tbsp dried oregano

Sea salt, to taste

Black pepper, to taste

Method

• Wash and dry kale.

• Remove leaves from stalks and slice into thin ribbons. Transfer to large mixing bowl.

• In small mixing bowl, add lemon juice, olive oil, oregano, salt, and pepper. Whisk thoroughly.

• Pour dressing over kale and massage for a minute with clean hands, kneading and rubbing.

• Toss in sliced cucumber and serve with extra fresh cracked black pepper, if desired.

IINsider Tip: Extra kale? Make Diana Chaplin's Kale and Turmeric Squash (V) (GF) *the same week, so you can use your kale twice. (See page 33.)*

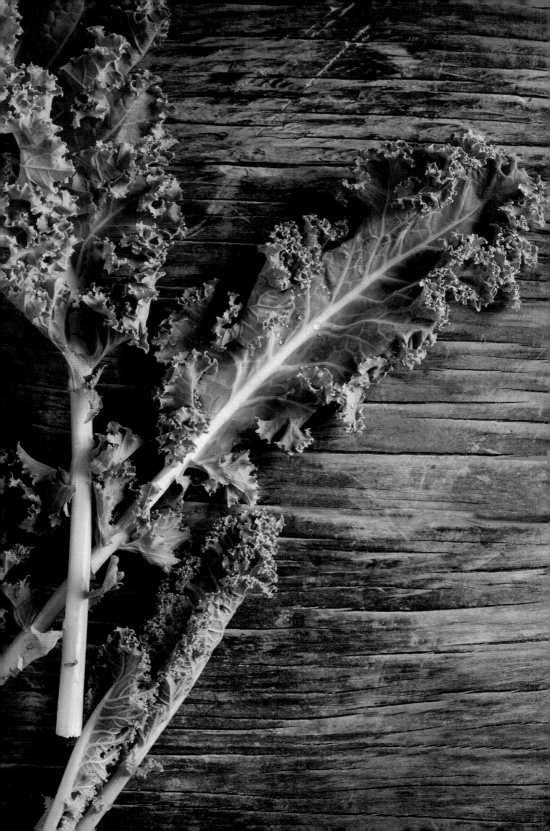

Kale and Turmeric Squash (V) (GF)

Diana Chaplin, Class of 2012

Prep time: 15 minutes
Cook time: 60 minutes

Ingredients
Serves 2–4

1 medium butternut squash, peeled and chopped into ¼-inch chunks

6 cups kale, chopped

2–3 stalks of scallions

¼ cup pine nuts

1 bulb of garlic

⅓ tsp ground turmeric

2 tbsps ghee or coconut oil

Sea salt, to taste

Black pepper, to taste

Olive oil

Method

- Melt ghee or coconut oil in pan, then add to large bowl with squash, garlic, sea salt, black pepper, and turmeric and mix thoroughly.

- Transfer to baking dish and bake at 350°F for 35–40 minutes, mixing occasionally so the squash cooks evenly.

- Spread out the pine nuts on a separate baking sheet and bake with sea salt on the top rack for 5 minutes, until golden brown.

- When squash mix is almost done, blanch kale for 2 minutes in water or vegetable stock, strain, and drizzle with olive oil.

- When ready to serve, combine squash mixture, kale, and pine nuts, and garnish with chopped scallions.

IINsider Tip: Have extra squash? Make Butternut Squash Soup with Crispy Sage (V) (GF) the same week. (See page 107.)

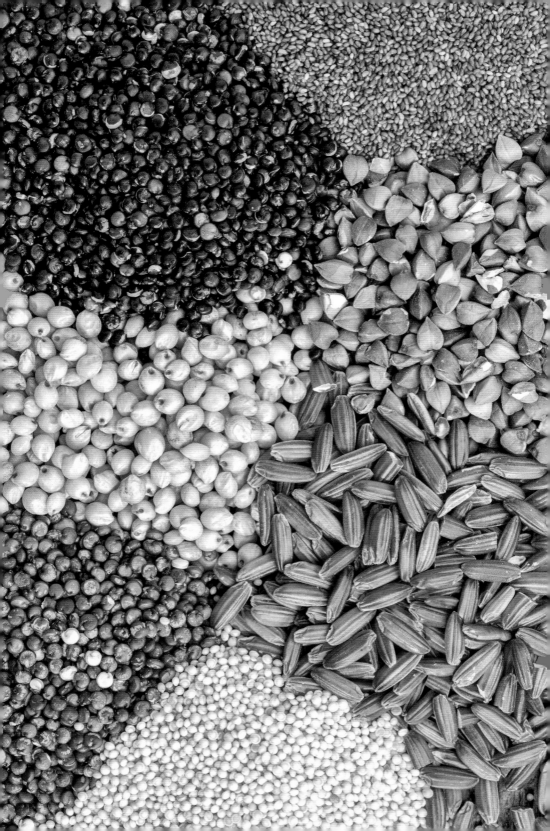

Chapter 2: Great Grains

Grains are the basis of many diets around the world. Whole grains provide slow-burning, high-quality energy and are packed with vital nutrients such as iron, vitamin E, and vitamin B-complex. Don't shy away from grains because they're carbohydrates—remember, they're not all created equal. What I mean by this is that refined carbohydrates like white rice and bread break down much faster in our bodies, playing havoc with our blood sugar levels. Have you ever experienced an energy crash? That was a probably a result of eating a refined-carb-rich meal. Compare this to complex carbohydrates like brown rice that are digested much slower and help maintain steady blood-sugar levels. These delicious and nutritious grains will keep you full and give your body the fuel it needs to thrive. In the Great Grains chapter, I'll teach you how to cook these staples for maximum nutrition and flavor.

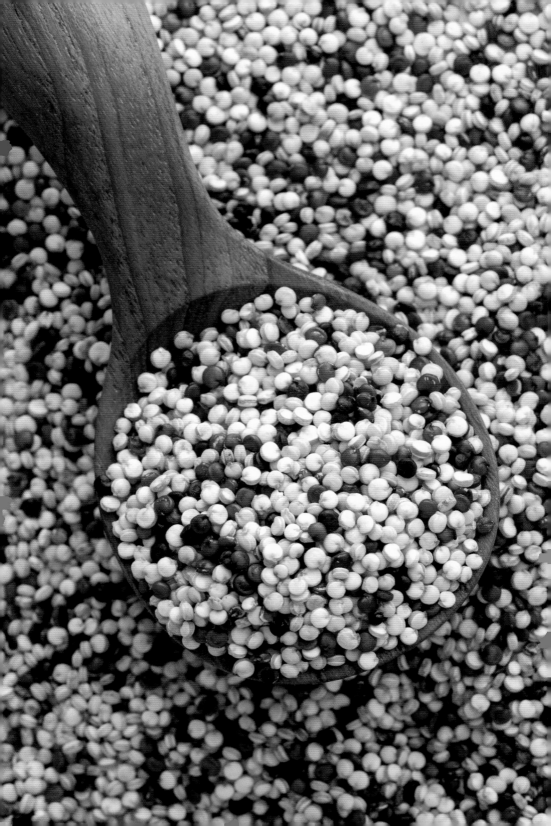

Classic Quinoa

Prep time: 10 minutes
Cook time: 35 minutes

Ingredients
Serves 5–6

1 cup dry quinoa

2 cups water

1 medium onion

1 carrot

2 stalks celery

1 bay leaf

1 tbsp olive oil

1 tsp sea salt

1 tsp black pepper

Method

• Rinse quinoa thoroughly in fine mesh strainer.

• Add to pot and cover with 2 cups water.

• Add a tablespoon of olive oil, bay leaf, and sea salt and bring to boil.

• Once it comes to a boil, turn to lowest heat, cover and cook for 20 minutes, until fluffy and translucent.

• Mince onion, carrot, and celery finely.

• In medium skillet, bring 1 tablespoon olive oil to medium heat.

• Add onions first and cook for 5 minutes, or until translucent.

• Add carrot and celery and cook for 5–7 more minutes.

• Add 1 cup cooked quinoa to pan along with sea salt and pepper and combine well.

• Store extra quinoa in container to use at another time.

IINsider Tip: Make Vegan Chili   *this week and serve it over your quinoa, or use your quinoa in the Hearty Mexican Bowl* . *(See pages 63 and 121.)*

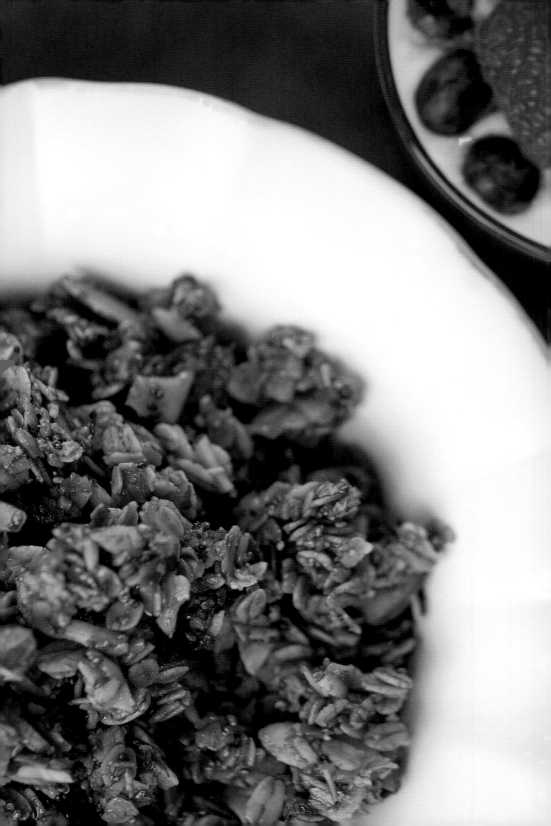

Superfood Granola with Goji Berries ⓥ 🄶🄵

Prep time: 10 hours
Cook time: 60 minutes

Ingredients
Serves 5–6

3 cups gluten-free rolled oats

½ cup sliced almonds

3 tbsps chia seeds

½ cup goji berries, soaked

¾ cup coconut palm sugar

¼ cup melted coconut oil

2 tbsps cinnamon

2 tsps fine Himalayan salt

Method

• Soak goji berries overnight. Strain and dry on paper towels.

• Preheat oven to 300°F.

• Combine all ingredients except goji berries in large bowl and mix thoroughly.

• Spread out in an even, ½-inch layer on a baking sheet and transfer to oven.

• Bake for 15 minutes, then stir, then return to oven for 10 minutes, then stir and return to oven again. Continue stirring every 10 minutes until granola is golden brown.

• Remove from oven and stir goji berries into mixture.

• Allow to cool for 15 minutes and store in a large glass jar and serve with coconut milk or yogurt.

IINsider Tip: Extra oats? Make Katie Flores' Pumpkin Pie Oatmeal   *this week. (See page 47.)*

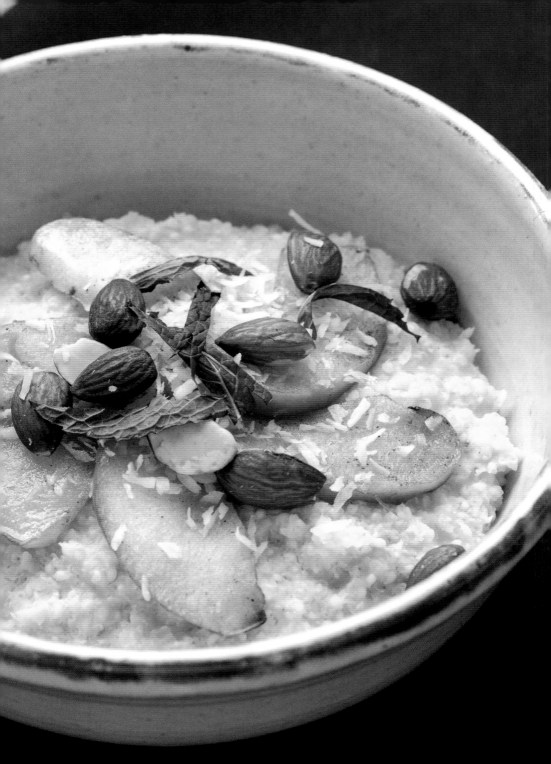

Millet Porridge with Caramelized Apples, Toasted Almonds, and Coconut (V) (GF)

Prep time: 5 minutes
Cook time: 25 minutes

Ingredients
Serves 5–6

1 cup dry millet

2 ½ cups water or milk of choice

1 apple

½ cup sliced almonds

½ cup coconut flakes

3 tbsps coconut oil or butter

Small pinch sea salt

Method

• Rinse millet in fine mesh strainer and transfer to medium pot.

• Add water or milk of choice and sea salt and bring to boil.

• Once it comes to a boil, reduce heat to lowest setting, cover, and simmer for 10 minutes.

• Toast sliced almonds and coconut flakes together in dry pan over medium heat for 5 minutes until fragrant and lightly browned. Set aside.

• Bring coconut oil or butter to medium heat and add apple.

• Allow to caramelize for 8 minutes, stirring only every few minutes.

• Serve millet topped with caramelized apples, almonds, and coconut.

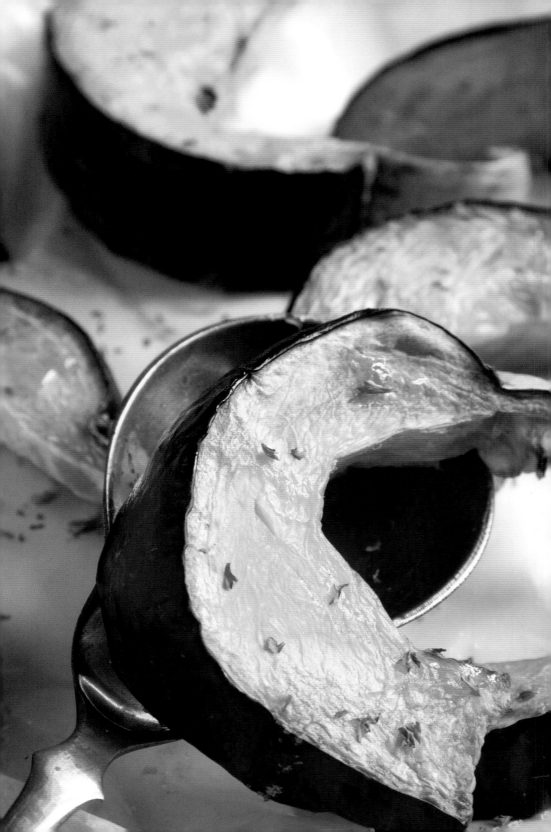

Warming Kasha with Winter Vegetables and Sage Glaze

Prep time: 15 minutes
Cook time: 65 minutes

Ingredients
Serves 5–6

1 cup dry kasha

2 cups water, vegetable stock, or chicken stock

1 medium onion

1 winter squash of choice

1 lb shiitake mushrooms

¼ cup fresh sage

2 tbsps maple syrup

2 tbsps butter or olive oil

1 tsp sea salt

1 tsp pepper

Method

• Preheat oven to 350°F.

• Trim squash ends, rinse, and pat dry.

• Cut in half, scoop out seeds, and pierce each side a few times with a fork.

• Rub with butter or olive oil.

• Set skin-side up on baking dish and bake for 30–45 minutes until very tender.

• While squash is cooking, bring liquid of choice to a boil in medium pot with sea salt.

• Rinse kasha in fine mesh strainer.

• Add kasha to boiling water and bring back to a boil; reduce heat and simmer for 10–12 minutes.

• Finely dice onion. Wash and pat dry mushrooms, then slice.

• In medium pan, bring butter or olive oil to medium heat.

• Sauté onion for 5 minutes, or until translucent.

• Add mushrooms and cook for 5 more minutes.

• Add cooked, diced squash.

• Add minced sage and 2 tablespoons maple syrup, along with salt and pepper to taste.

• Add kasha to pan and cook for 5 minutes.

• Serve as a side dish or simple, grounding main dish.

IINsider Tip: Got extra mushrooms? Make Sautéed Bok Choy with Shiitake Mushrooms and Shallots . *(See page 101.)*

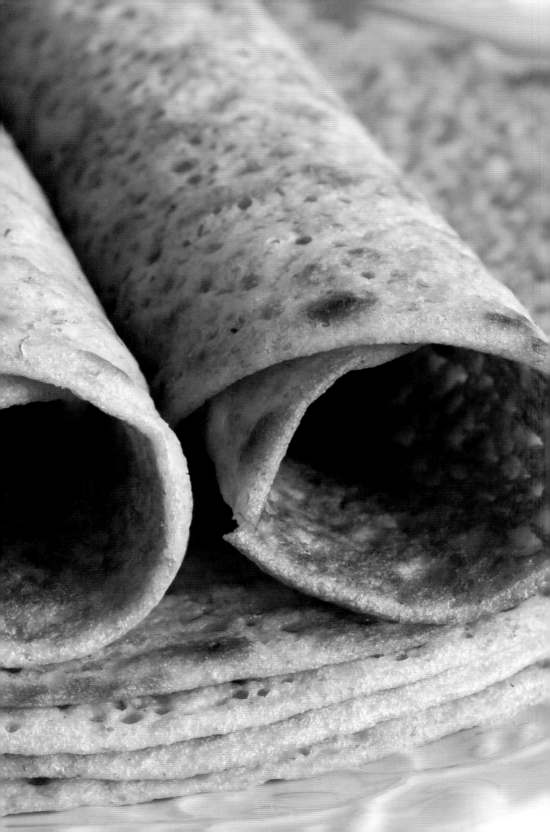

Savory Teff Crepes

Prep time: 10 minutes
Cook time: 30 minutes

Ingredients
Serves 3–4

½ cup teff flour

½ tsp sea salt

½ cup whole milk or full-fat coconut milk

1 egg

2 portobello mushrooms

1 medium yellow onion

½ tsp coriander

1 tbsp minced garlic

4 tbsps butter or olive oil

Additional sea salt, to taste

Black pepper, to taste

Method

• Combine teff flour with sea salt and whisk together in bowl.

• Combine milk of choice, egg, and melted butter or olive oil in separate larger bowl and whisk well.

• Add teff to liquid mixture and whisk well. Cover and set aside.

• Slice onion thin. Rinse mushrooms, trim, and slice thin.

• Add butter or olive oil to pan and bring to medium heat.

• Add onion and cook for 5 minutes, stirring frequently, until translucent.

• Add mushrooms and cook for 8 minutes, until wilted and combined.

• Add minced garlic, coriander, sea salt, and black pepper and cook for 5 more minutes.

• Transfer vegetable mixture to serving bowl.

• Bring two tablespoons butter or olive oil to medium-high heat in medium nonstick skillet.

• Pour crepe mixture into pan.

• Cook for 3 minutes on each side.

• Remove crepe and transfer to serving plate.

• Add ½ cup vegetable mixture in the center of each crepe and fold like a burrito or simply roll it up.

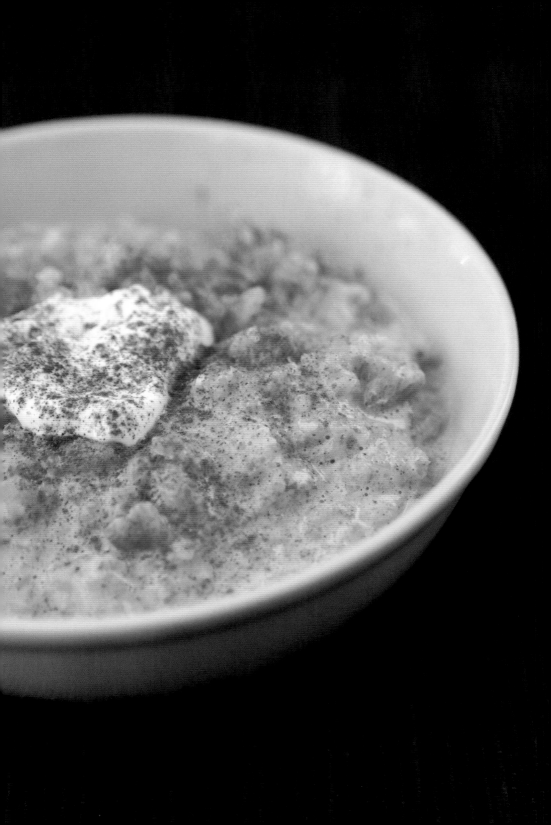

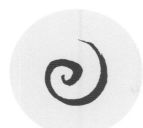

Pumpkin Pie Oatmeal

Katie Flores, Class of 2012

Prep time: 5 minutes
Cook time: 15 minutes

Ingredients
Serves 2–3

1 cup gluten-free rolled oats

1 cup pumpkin puree

1 cup coconut milk

2 cups water

1 tbsp vanilla extract

2 tsps pumpkin pie spice

¼ cup honey or maple syrup

Method

- Mix all ingredients except honey and pumpkin pie spice in saucepan.

- Cook on medium-low, mixing occasionally, until oatmeal reaches desired consistency.

- Transfer oatmeal to bowls.

- Stir in honey or maple syrup and sprinkle pumpkin pie spice on top.

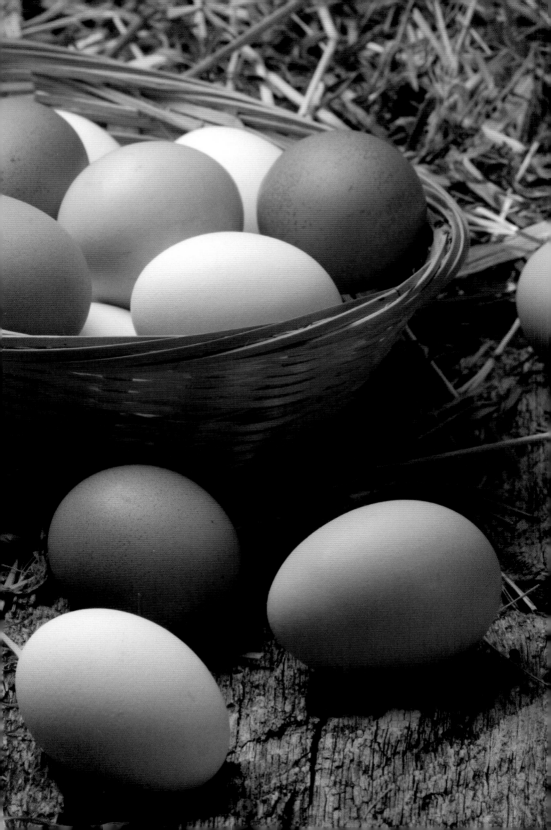

Chapter 3: Perfect Proteins

Protein is an essential food group and often the focus of meals. It's made up of amino acids, which are essential compounds our bodies need to function. In the Perfect Proteins chapter, I'll explore different types of protein that will provide your body with energy all day. Experiment with different sources and see which ones makes your body feel the most vibrant and energized. Try both plant and animal sources of protein and notice the difference in how you feel. How is your energy? How is your digestion? Remember to apply the principle of bio-individuality to protein: One person's food can be another person's poison.

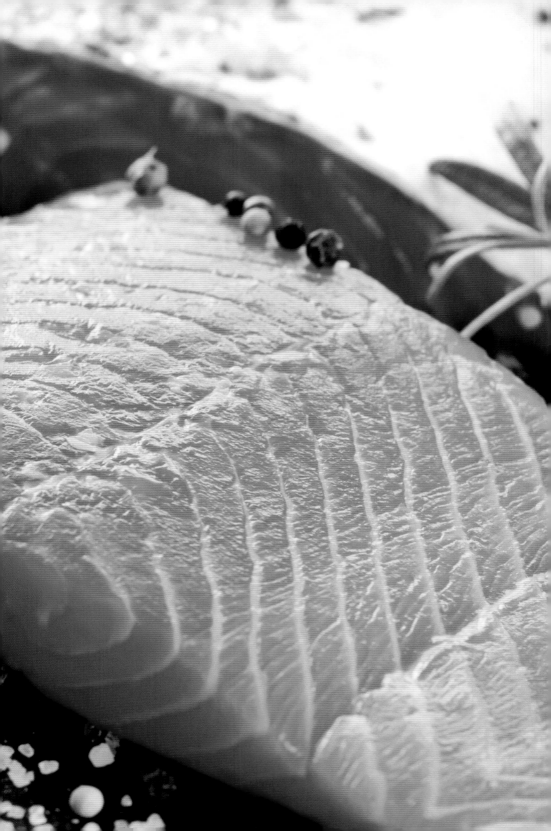

Sweet and Sour Glazed Salmon

Prep time: 20 minutes
Cook time: 10 minutes

Ingredients
Serves 4

4 wild salmon filets

¼ cup apple cider vinegar

¼ cup sesame oil

¼ cup tamari

1 tbsp lemon juice

1 tbsp honey

2 tbsps warm water

Method

• Set broiler to high heat.

• Rinse salmon filets, pat dry, and set aside in broiling dish.

• Allow to come to room temperature.

• Combine apple cider vinegar, sesame oil, tamari, and lemon juice in measuring cup and whisk well.

• Mix honey with warm water to create simple syrup and whisk into other liquid ingredients.

• Pour marinade over salmon and let sit for 10 minutes.

• Broil for 8 minutes, until flesh is opaque. Time will depend on thickness. For a 1-inch thick filet, 8 minutes will be perfect.

IINsider Tip: Leftover salmon? Make Salmon Burgers with Creamy Dill Sauce DF this week. (See page 109.)

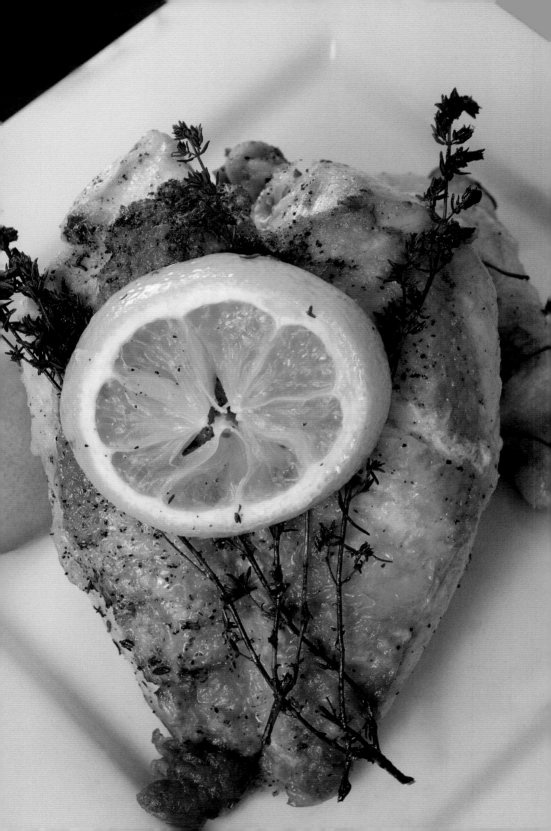

Roasted Chicken

Prep time: 15 minutes
Cook time: 80 minutes

Ingredients
Serves 6

4-lb whole chicken

1 medium yellow
onion

¼ lemon

1 bunch fresh
rosemary

1 bunch fresh thyme

2 tbsps butter, ghee, or
olive oil

Sea salt, to taste

Black pepper, to taste

Method

• Preheat oven to 400°F.

• Remove organs or have your butcher do it,
rinse chicken, pat dry, and place on roasting
pan.

• Rub chicken with melted butter, ghee, or olive
oil, and add sea salt and black pepper to taste.

• Chop onion and quarter lemon and stuff
internal cavity with onion, lemon, rosemary,
and thyme.

• Tie drumsticks together with string.

• Transfer roasting pan to oven rack and brown
for 15 minutes.

• Reduce heat to 350°F and roast for
approximately 65 minutes (about 20 minutes
per pound).

• Use a meat thermometer to ensure that thighs
are at 165–170°F, and check that juices run
clear from the breast.

• Serve with your favorite vegetables, grain,
and/or potatoes.

*IINsider Tip: Use leftover chicken pieces and the carcass to make Chicken and
Vegetable Soup* GF *this week. (See page 147.)*

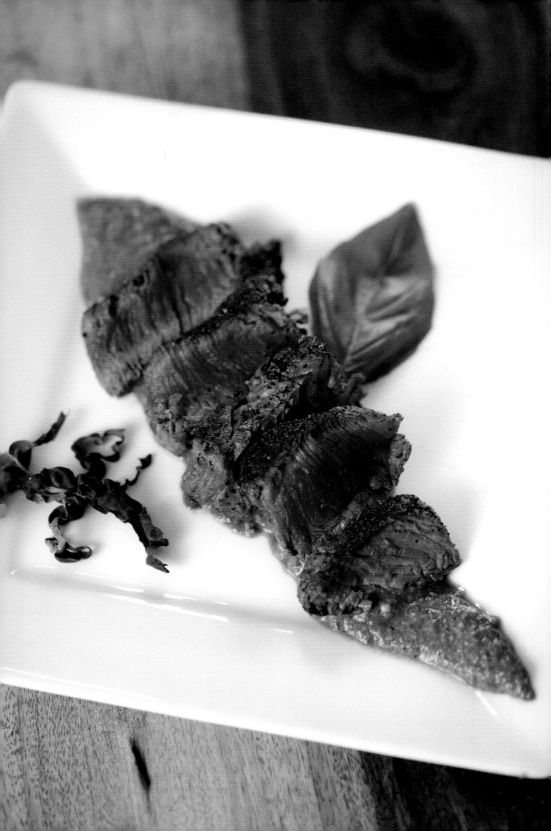

Seared Steak with Super Green Chimichurri GF DF

Prep time: 10 minutes
Cook time: 15 minutes

Ingredients
Serves 4

1 lb steak (grass-fed preferred)

5 large leaves kale

2 bunches basil

1 bunch parsley

1 clove garlic

¼ cup extra virgin olive oil

Sea salt, to taste

Black pepper, to taste

Method

• Wash and pat dry kale, basil, and parsley.

• Remove kale leaves from ribs.

• Chop kale, basil, and parsley and transfer to blender.

• Roughly chop garlic clove and add to blender along with olive oil, sea salt, and pepper.

• Pulse until you have a thick sauce. Set aside.

• Bring cast iron skillet or grill to high heat.

• Rub steak with sea salt and pepper and sear on high for 5–7 minutes on each side, depending on thickness and desired meat temperature.

• Serve steak with chimichurri and your favorite vegetable and/or starch.

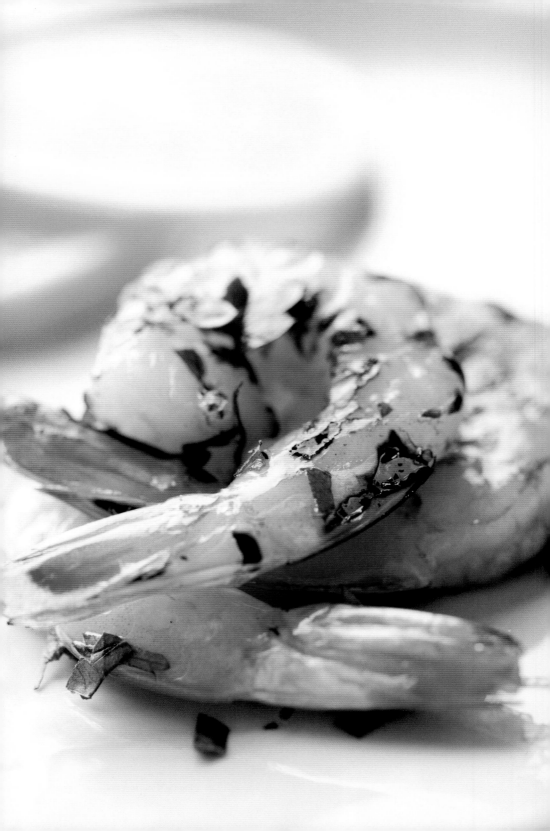

Grilled Shrimp

Prep time: 15 minutes
Cook time: 10 minutes

Ingredients
Serves 3–4

1 pound large shrimp

1 tbsp dried oregano

2 lemons

4 tbsps olive oil

Sea salt

Black pepper

Method

• Peel, devein, rinse, and pat dry shrimp and transfer to large mixing bowl.

• Sprinkle with dried oregano, olive oil, sea salt, and black pepper to taste.

• Grill outdoors for 3 minutes on each side or until cooked through, or sear in skillet or grill pan on the stove.

• Serve over your favorite salad.

• Finish with a squeeze of fresh lemon.

IINsider Tip: Leftover shrimp? Make Cauliflower Rice with Grilled Shrimp and Spicy Drizzle V GF *this week. (See page 141.)*

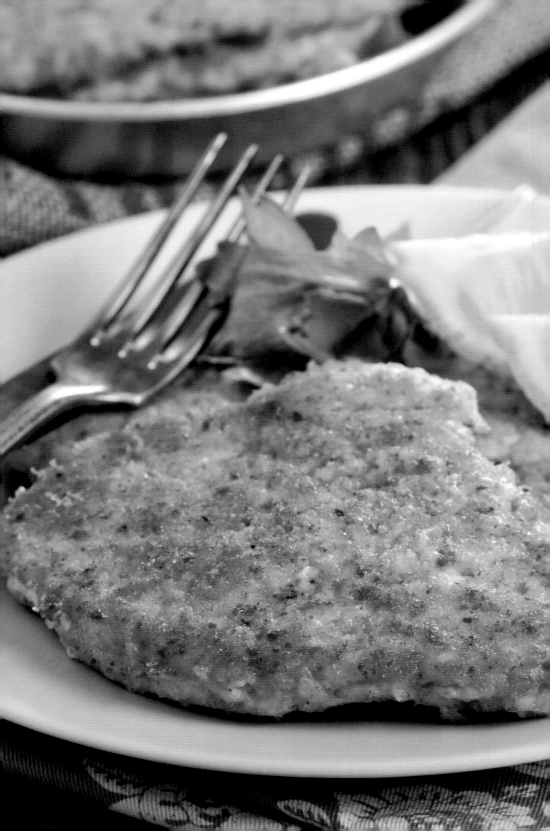

White Fish "Schnitzel"

Prep time: 15 minutes
Cook time: 15 minutes

Ingredients
Serves 3–4

1 lb firm wild white fish filets of choice, such as grouper, haddock, or cod

1 cup regular or gluten-free all-purpose flour

2 eggs or egg substitute

4 tbsps safflower oil

Sea salt, to taste

Black pepper, to taste

Lemon, for serving

Tartar sauce, for serving

Method

• Rinse fish filets, pat dry, and set on large plate.

• Combine flour with sea salt and pepper to taste in bowl. Beat eggs in another bowl.

• Add one tablespoon safflower oil to large nonstick skillet and bring to high heat.

• Coat fish filets in flour, then in egg, then in flour once more.

• Place fish in pan in one layer and sear for 4 minutes on each side or until flesh is translucent.

• Set cooked fish on a plate lined with a paper towel to absorb excess oil.

• Add more oil to pan as needed as you cook the fish in batches.

• Serve with a squeeze of lemon and your favorite high-quality tartar sauce.

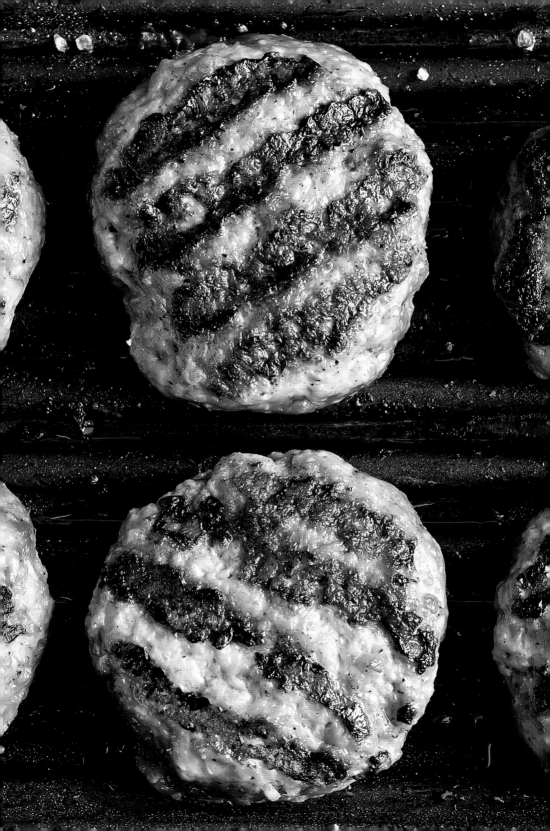

Turkey Burgers

Prep time: 10 minutes
Cook time: 30 minutes

Ingredients
Serves 4

1 lb lean, organic ground turkey

1 medium red onion

8 large portobello caps

1 avocado

4 tbsps organic ketchup

4 tbsps olive oil

Sea salt, to taste

Black pepper, to taste

Method

• Form turkey into four patties and grill or sear on high heat in olive oil for 6 minutes on each side or until cooked through. Let rest for 5 minutes.

• Bring one tablespoon olive oil to medium heat in nonstick skillet.

• Slice onions thin and cook for 5 minutes until caramelized.

• Add sea salt and pepper to taste in the last minute of cooking. Set onions aside.

• Rinse, pat dry, and rub portobello caps with 1 tablespoon olive oil.

• Grill for 3 minutes on each side or sear over high heat in pan with olive oil.

• Assemble turkey burgers by placing on top of one mushroom cap and garnishing with caramelized onions, sliced avocado, sea salt and pepper to taste, and organic ketchup.

• Top with another mushroom cap to complete the "bun."

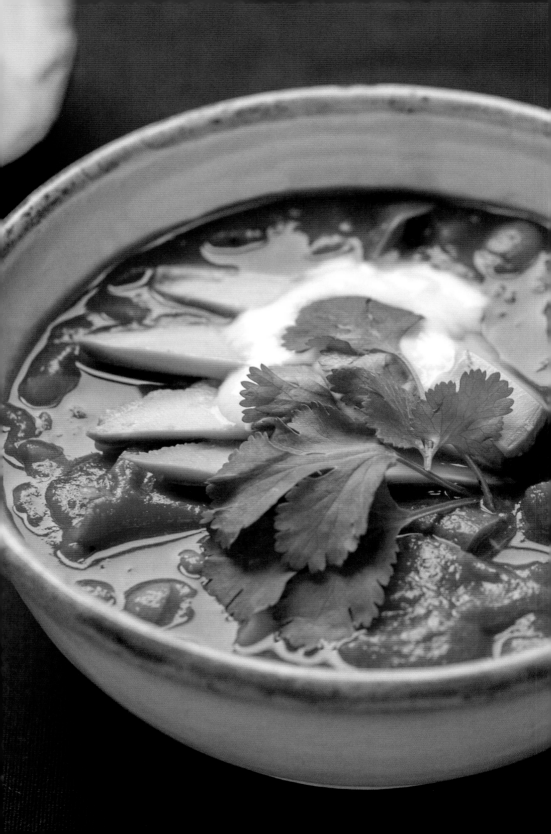

Vegan Chili Ⓥ GF

Prep time: 15 minutes
Cook time: 75 minutes

Ingredients
Serves 6–8

2 cups pinto beans

2 cups diced tomatoes

6 cups vegetable stock

1 large yellow onion

1 yellow pepper

1 red pepper

1 green pepper

1 tbsp ground cumin

¼ cup fresh cilantro

3 tbsps olive oil

1 tsp maple syrup

Sea salt, to taste

Black pepper, to taste

Brown rice or quinoa
(optional)

Method

- Bring olive oil to medium heat in heavy-bottom pot.

- Slice onions and cook for 5 minutes, or until caramelized.

- Slice peppers and add, cooking for 5 more minutes.

- Add tomatoes and beans and cook for 5 minutes, combining well.

- Add cumin, maple syrup, sea salt, and black pepper and stir well.

- Pour 6 cups vegetable stock over top, turn to high heat, and bring to boil.

- Once stock comes to a boil, reduce to low heat, cover, and simmer for an hour.

- Wash cilantro, pat dry, chop, and use as garnish.

- Serve as-is or over brown rice or quinoa.

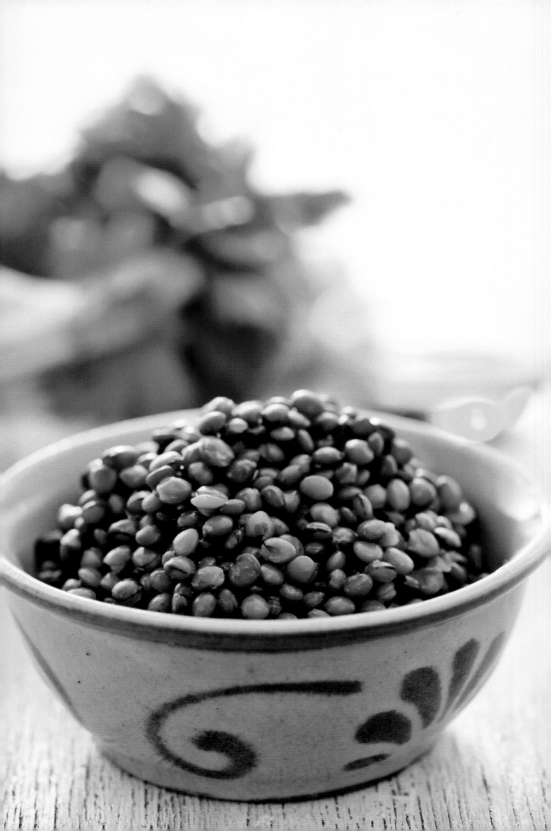

Grad Feature

Spaghetti and Lentil "Meatballs"

Nicole Smith, Class of 2013

Prep time: 20 minutes
Cook time: 50 minutes

Ingredients
Serves 4

1 cup dry lentils

½ cup gluten-free breadcrumbs

1 package brown rice pasta

1 jar pasta sauce

2 cups vegetable broth or water

1 egg

2 cloves garlic

1 tsp dried oregano

1 tsp sea salt

1 tsp pepper

Grated Parmesan cheese to top (optional)

Method

- Preheat oven to 350°F.

- Bring the vegetable broth and lentils to a boil and cook over medium heat for 15–20 minutes or until lentils are tender.

- Combine egg, sea salt, pepper, garlic, and oregano in a food processor.

- When the lentils are done, add those too. Pulse until blended well.

- Fold in the breadcrumbs.

- If the mixture is too dry, add another egg. If it's too wet, add more breadcrumbs (you want it a little more on the wet side).

- Line a cookie sheet with parchment paper.

- Using wet hands, roll the mixture into 1-inch balls. You can also use a small ice cream scoop. Place on sheet.

- Bake the lentil "meatballs" for 20 minutes or until golden brown.

- While they're baking, cook your pasta according to the directions on the package.

- Heat the pasta sauce.

- Drain pasta and divide into bowls. Top with a few "meatballs" and sauce.

IINsider Tip: Leftover lentils? Make Sarah Sunshine Kagan's Lentil Mushroom Burgers V GF *this week. (See page 111.)*

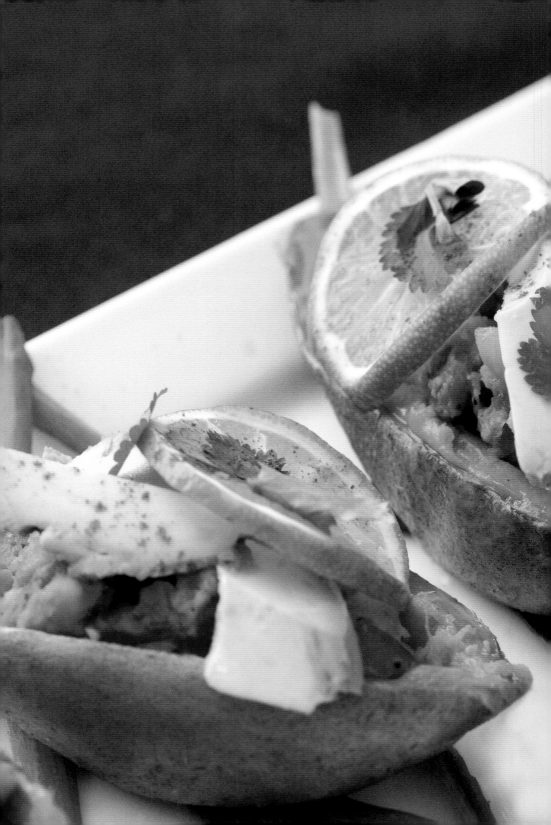

Sides and Shares

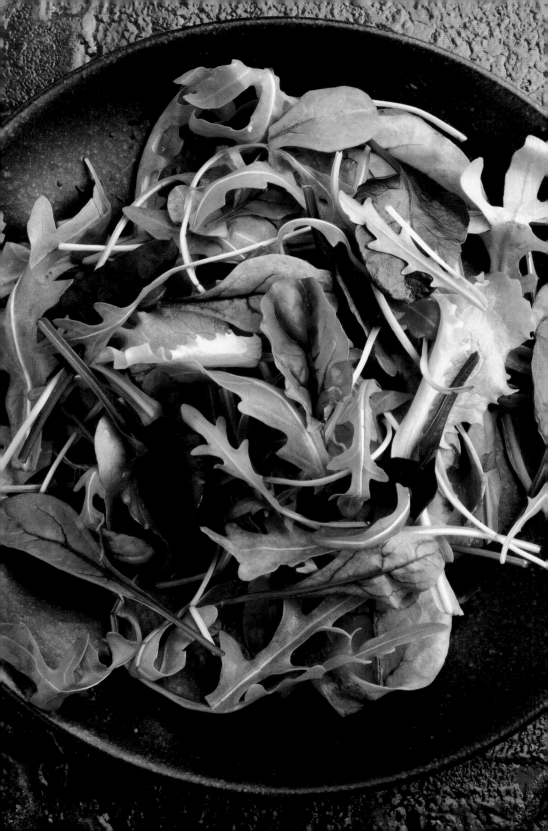

Chapter 4: Appetizers

In the Appetizers chapter, you'll learn how to make a great first impression. They say first impressions are everything, after all. If that's the case, you'll want to impress your loved ones with healthy and delicious starters. Whether you're breaking out your special serving dishes or just making yourself a midday snack, these recipes will nourish your soul and provide key vitamins and minerals.

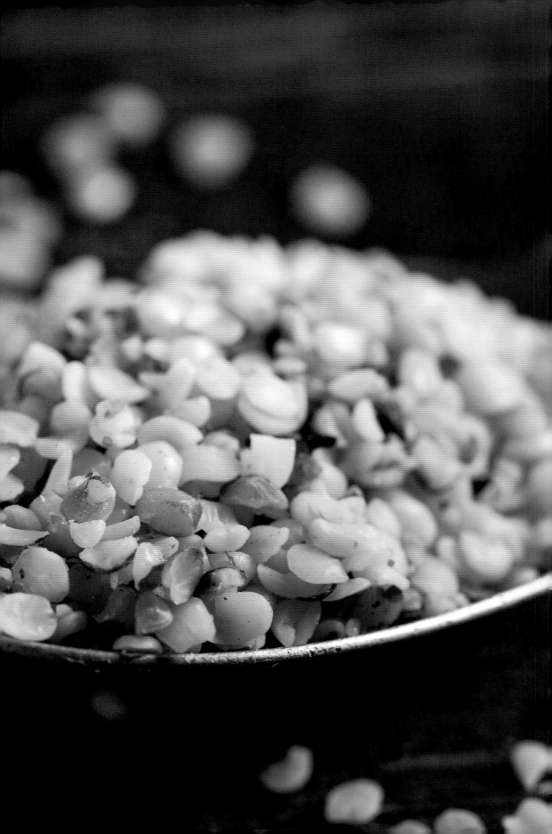

Hemp Seed Hummus

Prep time: 15 minutes
Cook time: 0 minutes

Ingredients
Serves 6–8

2 cups cooked
chickpeas

¼ cup tahini

¼ cup hemp seeds

¼ cup extra virgin
olive oil

¼ cup water, or more,
as needed

2 garlic cloves

Juice of 1 lemon

Sea salt, to taste

Method

• Slice garlic and combine all ingredients in
  blender.

• Blend until smooth, adding more olive oil
  and/or water as needed.

• Garnish with more hemp seeds and serve
  with your favorite vegetables.

IINsider Tip: Leftover chickpeas? Make Falafels with Tzatziki VG *this week.
(See page 123.)*

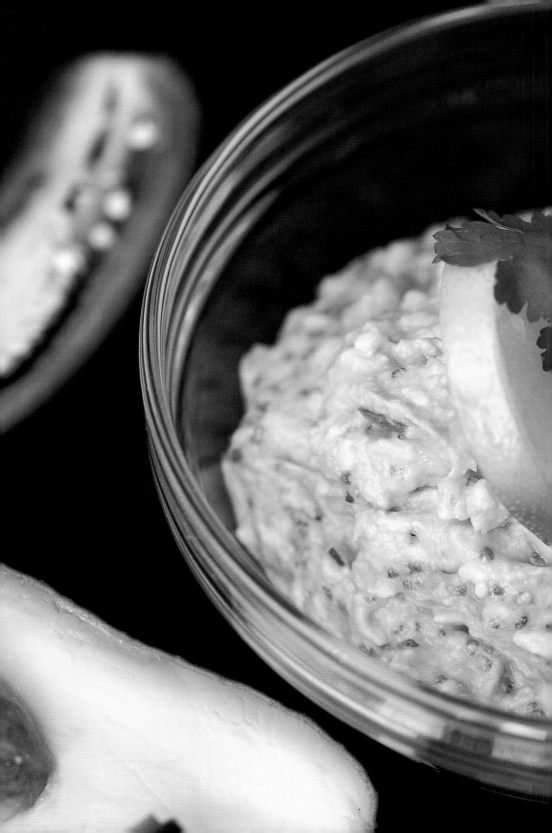

Superfood Guacamole

Prep time: 15 minutes
Cook time: 0 minutes

Ingredients
Serves 5–6

3 avocados

1 small red onion

1 jalapeño pepper

Juice of 3 limes

½ cup cilantro, chopped

½ cup chia seeds, soaked

Sea salt, to taste

Method

• Halve and score avocadoes and scoop out into bowl.

• Finely dice red onion, jalapeño, and cilantro and add to bowl.

• Add lime juice, soaked chia seeds, and sea salt.

• Mash all ingredients until creamy with small chunks.

• Serve with your favorite vegetables or corn tortilla chips.

IINsider Tip: Extra guacamole? Make the Hearty Mexican Bowl V GF *or Grilled Tempeh Collard "Tacos"* V GF *this week. (See pages 121 and 131.) Leftover avocado? Make Eileen Z. Fuentes's Grilled Pineapple, Watercress, and Avocado Salad* V GF. *(See page 81.)*

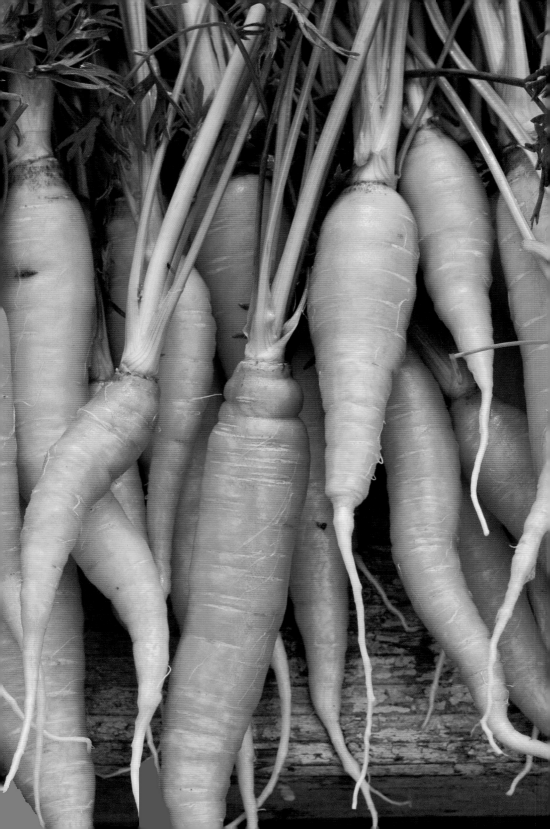

Carrot-Ginger Soup

Prep time: 10 minutes
Cook time: 40 minutes

Ingredients
Serves 4

6–7 large carrots

1 medium onion

½-inch knob of ginger

3 cups vegetable stock

3 tbsps extra virgin
coconut oil

Sea salt, to taste

Method

- Wash and pat dry carrots and ginger.

- Chop carrots and onions.

- Grate ginger.

- Bring coconut oil to medium heat in medium-large pot.

- Sauté onions until translucent but not browned.

- Add ginger and sea salt and cook for another 2 minutes.

- Add carrots and cook for 5 minutes.

- Cover with 3 cups water.

- Bring to a boil, then reduce to low heat and simmer for 20–25 minutes, until carrots are tender and soup is fragrant.

- Turn off heat; let sit for 10–15 minutes to cool.

- Then transfer soup to blender and blend until smooth and creamy. You could also use an immersion blender directly in the pot.

Options

- Garnish with cilantro

- Add 1 teaspoon curry powder or cinnamon

- For a creamier version, add ¼ cup full-fat coconut milk to blender

IINsider Tip: Leftover carrots? Make the Rooted juice V GF *this week.*
(See page 161.)

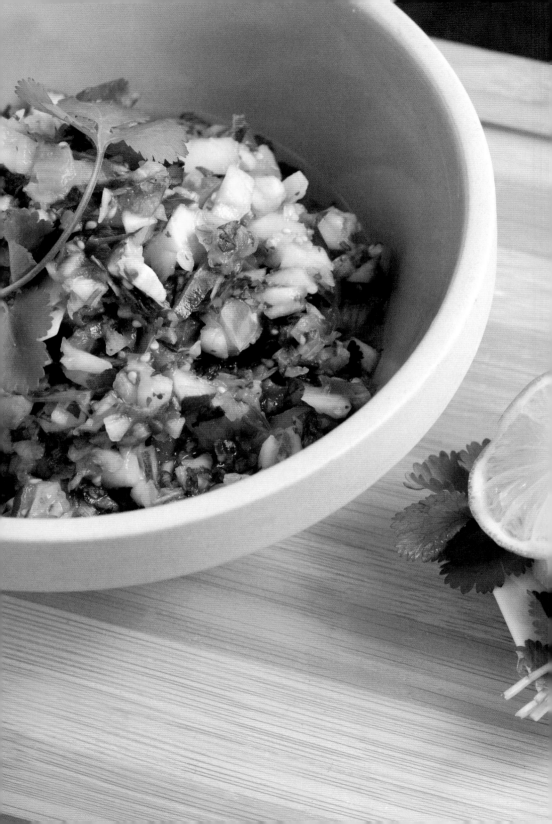

Peach Salsa with Jicama Chips

Prep time: 30 minutes
Cook time: 0 minutes

Ingredients
Serves 6–8

3 large jicama roots

3 peaches

2 medium heirloom tomatoes

1 medium red onion

1 jalapeño

Juice of 5 limes

¼ cup minced cilantro

Sea salt, to taste

Black pepper, to taste

Method

• Wash and pat dry peaches, tomatoes, jalapeño, limes, and cilantro.

• De-pit peaches and chop peaches and tomatoes.

• Mince onion, jalapeño, and cilantro.

• Combine all ingredients in large bowl and mix well.

• Transfer to container or glass jar and refrigerate for 15 minutes or longer to allow flavors to combine.

• When ready to serve, peel and slice jicama root thin, squeeze on lime, and serve with salsa.

IINsider Tip: Extra tomatoes? Make my Traditional Bulgarian Salad V GF *with optional feta cheese this week. (See page 79.) Extra salsa? Make my Hearty Mexican Bowl* V GF *this week. (See page 121.)*

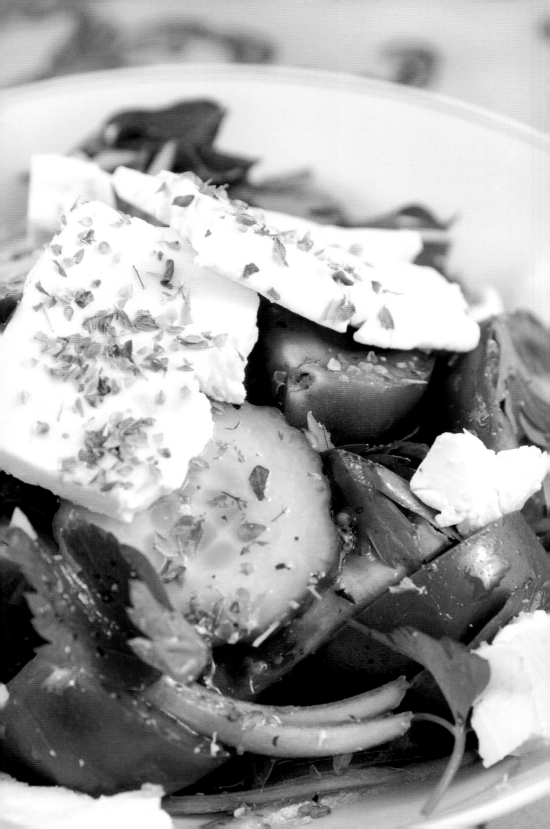

Traditional Bulgarian Salad

Prep time: 15 minutes
Cook time: 0 minutes

Ingredients
Serves 4–6

1 English cucumber

5 tomatoes

3 green onions, sliced

¼ cup chopped fresh parsley

½ cup extra virgin olive oil

¼ cup ume plum vinegar or red wine vinegar

Sea salt, to taste

Black pepper, taste

½ cup crumbled feta cheese (optional)

Method

• Wash and pat dry cucumber, tomatoes, and parsley. If not organic or if you prefer a milder flavor, peel cucumbers.

• Slice the cucumber into rounds. Dice tomatoes, green onions, and parsley.

• Transfer all ingredients to large bowl and toss with olive oil, vinegar, sea salt, and black pepper.

• If desired, top with feta cheese and serve.

IINsider Tip: Extra cucumbers? Make my Pure Sunshine Green Juice   *this week. (See page 157.)*

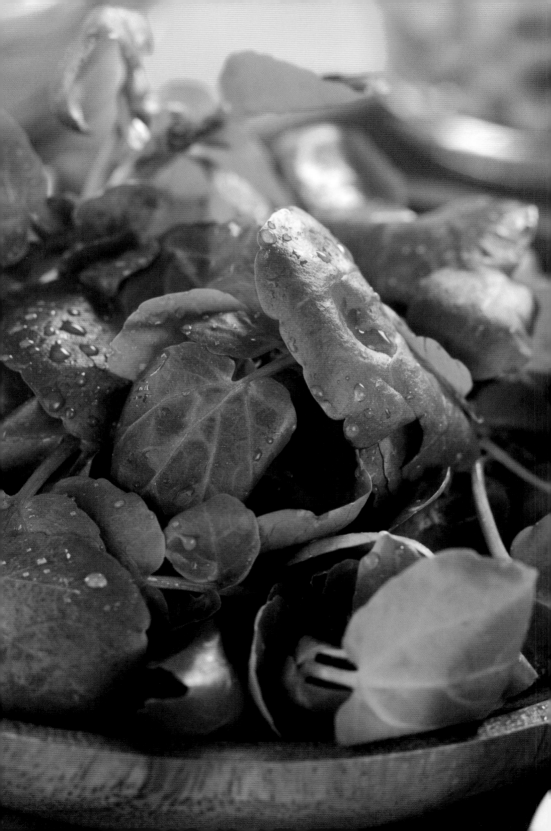

Grilled Pineapple, Watercress, and Avocado Salad

Eileen Z. Fuentes, Class of 2011

Prep time: 15 minutes
Cook time: 10 minutes

Ingredients
Serves 4–6

1 bunch watercress

1 pineapple, peeled, cored, and cut into 1-inch thick slices

1 avocado

1 small red onion

2 garlic cloves, finely chopped

Drizzle of extra virgin olive oil

Drizzle of apple cider vinegar or fresh lime juice

Sprinkle of coconut palm sugar

Ground cumin, to taste

Himalayan salt, to taste

Black pepper, taste

Method

- Rinse watercress in colander. Discard any yellow leaves. Pat dry with paper towel or spin dry.

- Set stovetop grill or barbecue to medium-high heat.

- Place the pineapple slices on baking sheet and sprinkle coconut palm sugar over them.

- Transfer pineapple to grill and cook for 5–7 minutes on each side, until golden brown.

- While pineapple is grilling, place garlic, olive oil, apple cider vinegar or lime juice, cumin, salt, and pepper in a small bowl and whisk to combine. Taste for seasoning. Set aside.

- De-pit and cut avocado into 1-inch cubes.

- Place the watercress in a medium bowl and toss with half the dressing, then arrange on a platter.

- Add the pineapple and avocado to the same bowl and toss with the rest of the dressing.

- Mound the pineapple and avocado over the watercress. Garnish with slivers of red onion and serve immediately.

IINsider Tip: Extra pineapple? Make my Pineapple-Lemon Zinger   *this week. (See page 163.)*

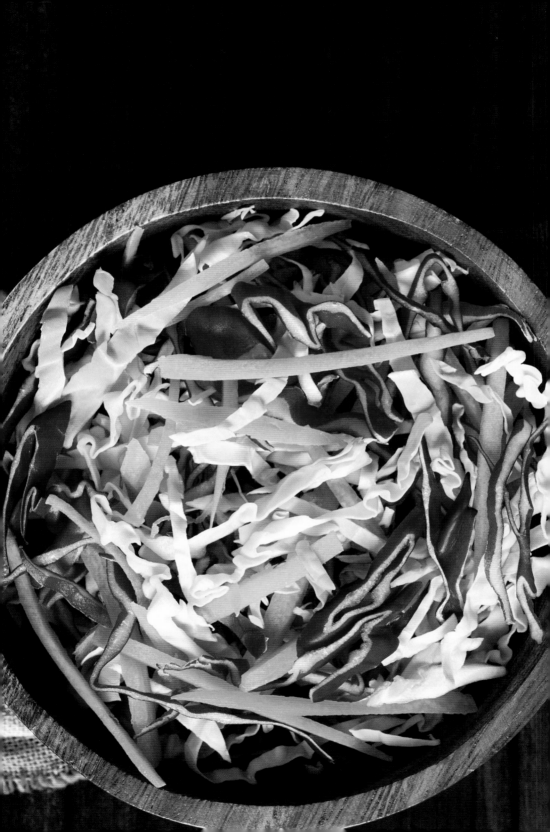

Chapter 5: Side Dishes

In the Side Dishes chapter, I'll teach you how to create beautiful small dishes that can be eaten alongside a main or on their own for a light meal or snack. Sides are a great way to complement your healthy main dish and add even more nutrients to your meal. In fact, side dishes, especially those with fermented and cultured ingredients, can help support your digestion throughout a meal. Try one of these quick, flavorful bites to complement your centerpiece and make your meal even healthier and more satisfying.

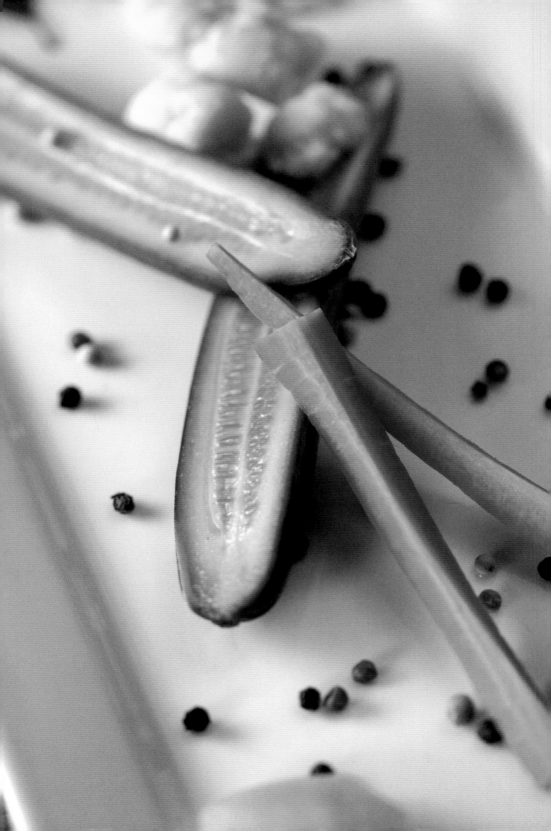

Mixed Pickles

Prep time: 10 minutes
Cook time: 3 days

Ingredients
Serves 8–10

1 cup sliced carrots

1 cup sliced cucumbers

1 cup cauliflower, cut
into small florets

4 cups warm filtered
water

1 bay leaf

2 tbsps sea salt

1 tsp black
peppercorns

Method

• Combine water, sea salt, and peppercorns
well.

• Add all vegetables to large glass jar along with
bay leaf.

• Cover with salt-water mixture, leaving 1-inch
of space at the top of the jar.

• Cover jar tightly and let sit at room
temperature, out of the fridge.

• Once a day, open the jar to release air and
taste the pickles.

• When they've reached your desired taste,
transfer them to the refrigerator, which slows
down the fermentation process.

*IINsider Tip: Extra cauliflower? Make Andrea Saunder's Marinated Cauliflower
Salad*   *this week. (See page 95.)*

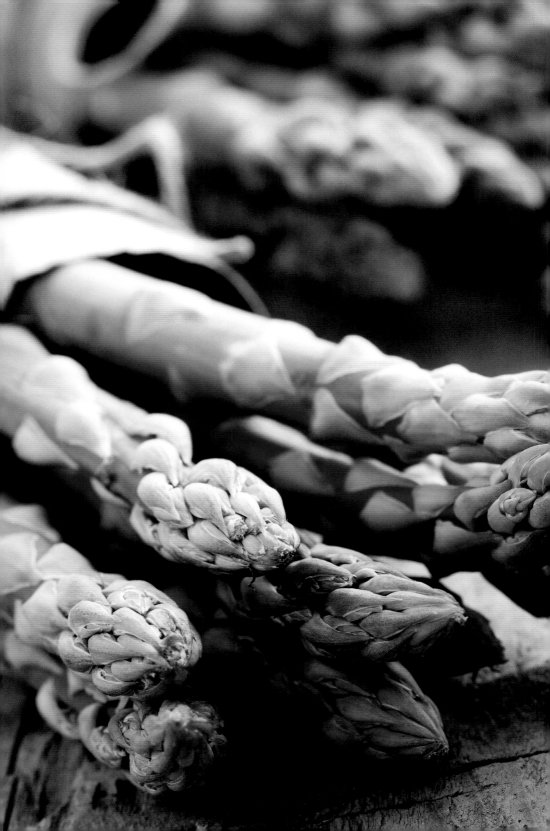

Grilled Asparagus with Creamy Sweet Potato Sauce and Crispy Rosemary (V) (GF)

Prep time: 4 hours
Cook time: 20 minutes

Ingredients
Serves 2

1 bunch fresh asparagus

1 sweet potato

½ cup cashews

¼ cup coconut milk

1 bunch rosemary

Sea salt, to taste

Black pepper, to taste

Method

• Soak cashews in filtered water for 4 hours or overnight.

• Rinse asparagus and sweet potatoes and cube sweet potatoes. Break off tough asparagus ends.

• Bring 3 cups of salted water to a boil and add the sweet potatoes first, then the asparagus.

• Remove asparagus after 3 minutes and transfer to plate.

• Allow sweet potato to simmer for 5 more minutes or until tender. Transfer to plate.

• Add sweet potato, soaked cashews, coconut milk, sea salt, and pepper to blender and blend on high until creamy. Add water if too thick.

• Bring olive oil to medium-high heat in pan and sear asparagus for 3–5 minutes on each side, until slightly charred.

• Rinse and pat dry rosemary and add to pan after you remove asparagus.

• Cook rosemary for a minute or less, just until crispy but not burnt.

• Ladle sauce over asparagus and top with rosemary.

IINsider Tip: Extra sweet potatoes? Make My Mom's Sweet Potato and Thyme (V) (GF) *this week. (See page 91.)*

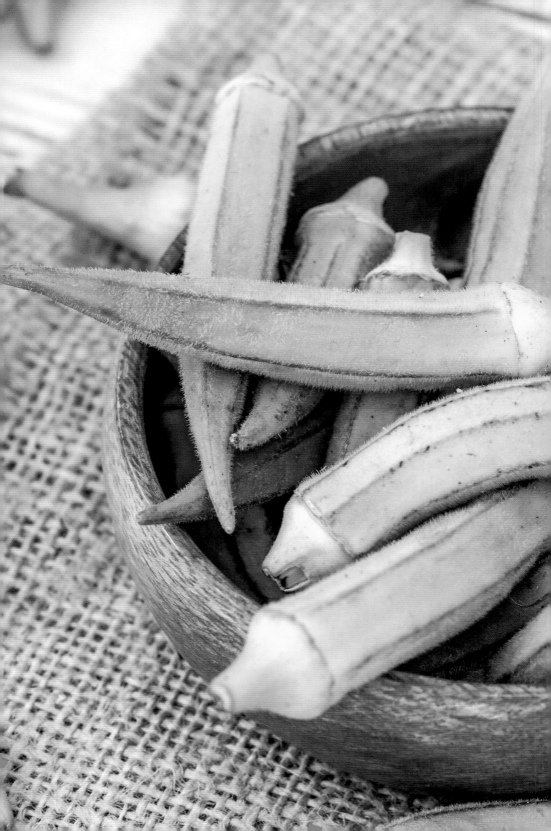

Roasted Okra and Onion

Prep time: 10 minutes
Cook time: 15 minutes

Ingredients
Serves 4

1 lb okra pods, trimmed and cut in half lengthwise

1 small sweet yellow onion, sliced in crescents

2 tbsps extra virgin olive oil

¼ cup chopped fresh basil and mint

Sea salt, to taste

Black pepper, to taste

Method

• Preheat oven to 400°F.

• Wash and pat dry okra, basil, and mint.

• Combine okra and onion in a bowl with olive oil, sea salt, and black pepper.

• Toss well to coat.

• Roast in oven 10 minutes or until tender.

• Toss with fresh basil and mint and serve.

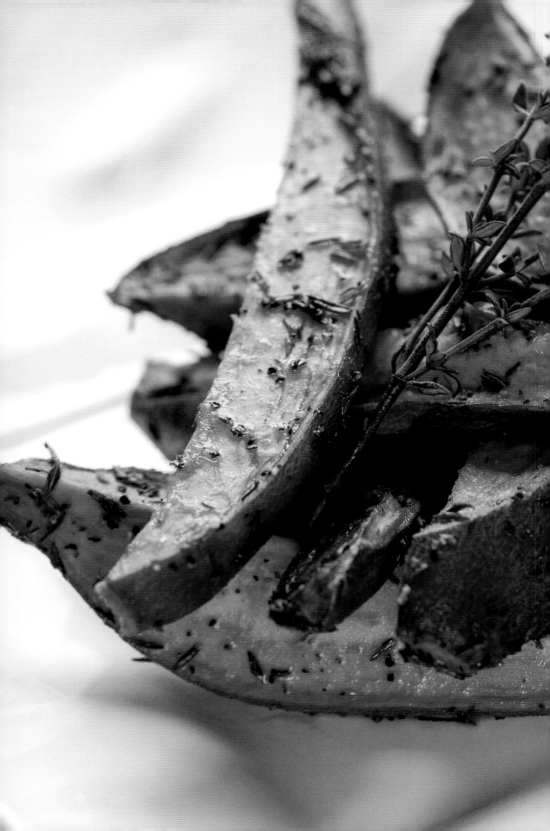

My Mom's Sweet Potato and Thyme ⓥ ⒼⒻ

Prep time: 10 minutes
Cook time: 30 minutes

Ingredients
Serves 4–6

4 medium-large sweet potatoes

3 tbsps fresh or dried thyme

3 tbsps extra virgin olive oil or melted ghee

Sea salt, to taste

Black pepper, to taste

Method

• Preheat oven to 350°F.

• Wash sweet potatoes, pat dry, and peel if not organic.

• Chop into ½-inch cubes.

• Toss in large mixing bowl with olive oil or melted ghee, thyme, sea salt, and black pepper.

• Spread out on baking sheet and roast for 20–30 minutes until tender and golden-brown.

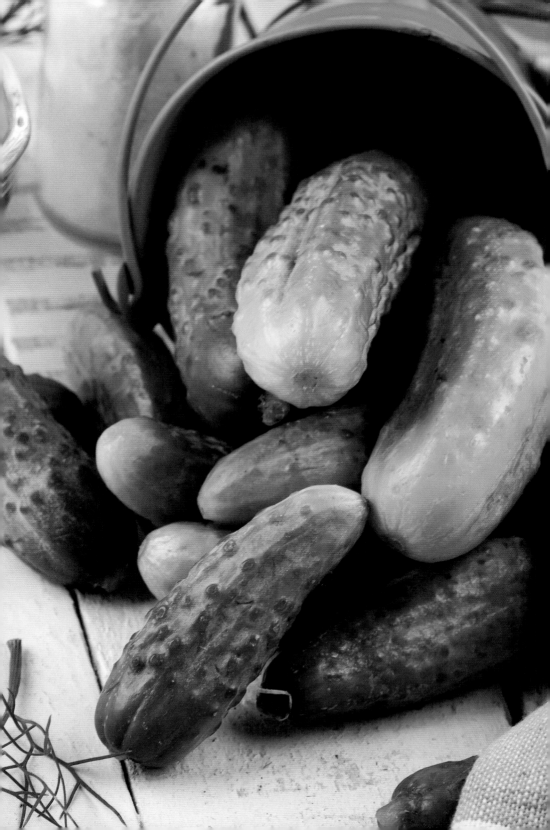

Cucumber-Dill Salad with Grilled Pita VG

Prep time: 15 minutes
Cook time: 5 minutes

Ingredients
Serves 3–4

2 large English cucumbers

1 bunch dill

2 cloves garlic, minced

Juice of 3 lemons

¼ cup plain Greek yogurt

3 tbsps olive oil

3–4 whole wheat pitas

Sea salt, to taste

Black pepper, to taste

Method

• Wash cucumbers, pat dry, peel if not organic and/or if you prefer a milder flavor, and dice into cubes. Transfer to medium bowl.

• Wash dill, pat dry, and mince.

• Add dill, olive oil, Greek yogurt, lemon juice, sea salt, and black pepper to cucumbers and toss well.

• Bring grill or pan to medium-high heat.

• Brush pitas with olive oil and grill for 3–4 minutes on each side until toasted.

• Slice pitas into triangles and serve with cucumber salad.

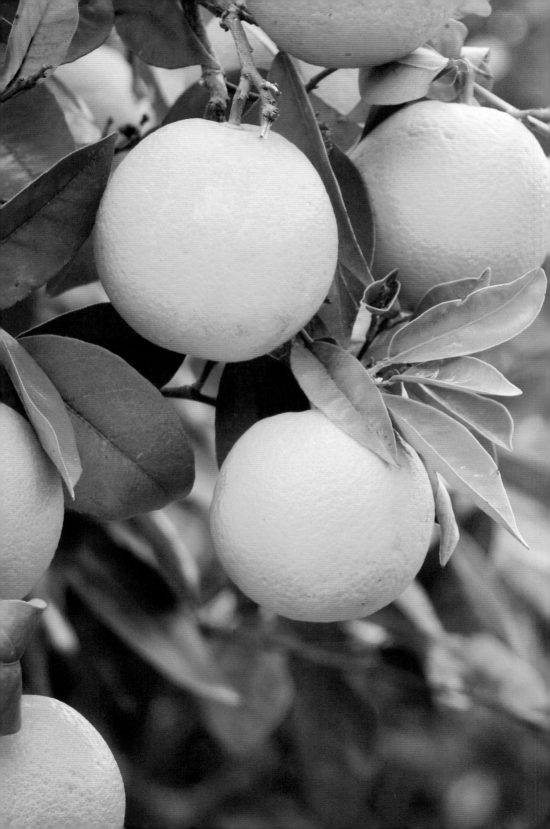

Marinated Cauliflower Salad Ⓥ ⒼⒻ

Andrea Saunder, Class of 2013

Prep time: 20 minutes
Cook time: 4 hours

Ingredients

Serves 2–4

4 raw cauliflower florets, cut into bite-sized pieces

1 large orange

1 apple, cored and chopped into bite-sized pieces

1 shallot, finely sliced

1 clove garlic, finely sliced

4 tbsps olive oil

Juice of 1 lemon

Handful of walnuts, roughly chopped

Handful of fresh herbs of your choice

Method

- Peel orange and remove the pith and seeds. Do this in a strainer, over a large bowl to catch all the juice. Roughly chop the flesh into bite-sized pieces and add back to the bowl.

- Add all remaining ingredients to bowl and mix, making sure oil and citrus juices combine with all other ingredients.

- Cover bowl and allow to marinate for at least 4 hours and up to 2 days. If marinating for use the next day, store in fridge.

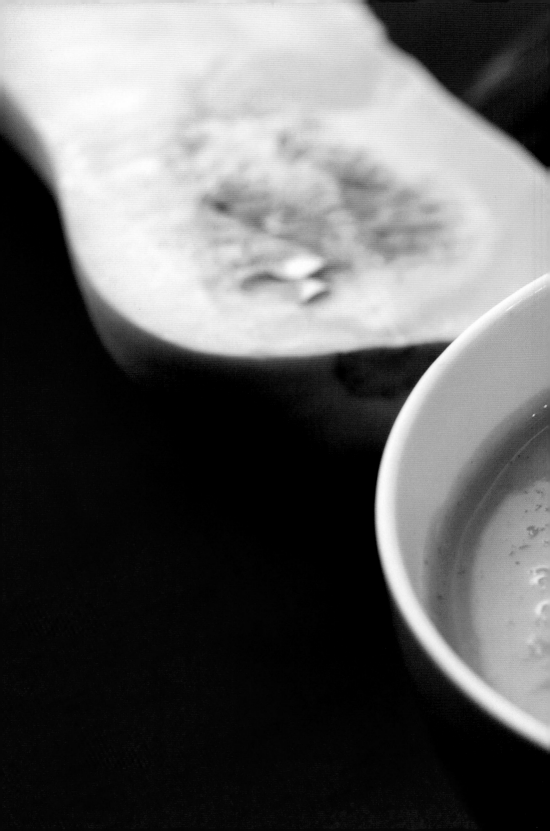

Freedom Favorites

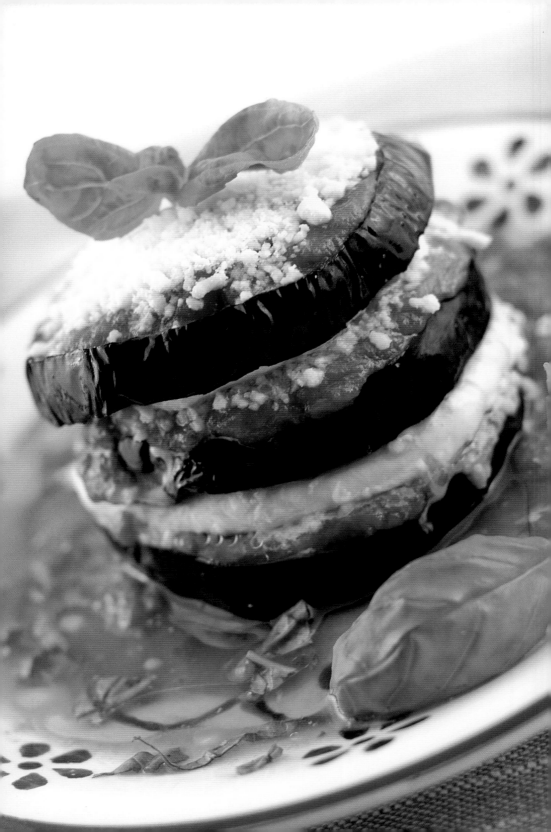

Chapter 6: Dairy-Free

Many people avoid dairy because they don't digest it well and feel more energized when they eliminate it from their diets. A dairy-free diet may help people clear up issues with mucus and congestion. If you've realized that a dairy-free diet works best for you but you miss the comforting taste and texture, try these recipes. The Dairy-Free chapter might make you realize you don't need dairy and can still enjoy great flavors, or you might realize you love dairy and your body can handle it—both are okay. Feel free to use the recipes in this chapter to experiment with going dairy-free.

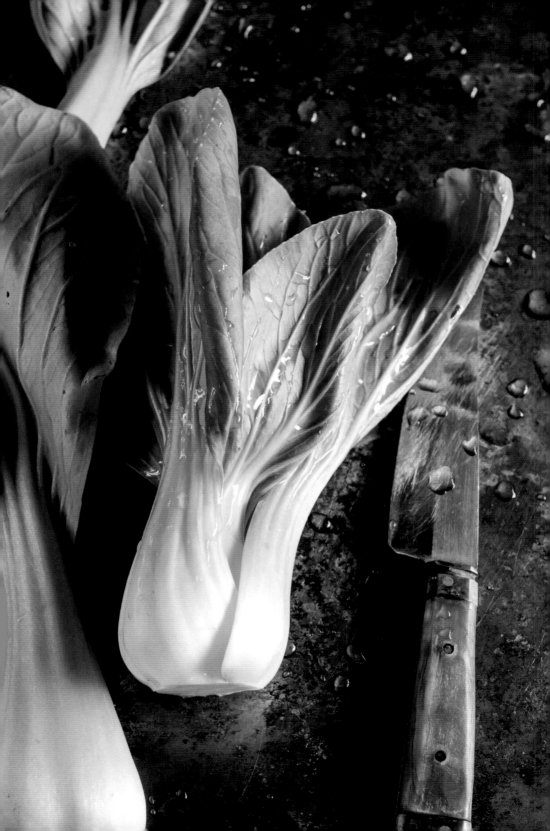

Sautéed Bok Choy with Shiitake Mushrooms and Shallots (V) (GF)

Prep time: 10 minutes
Cook time: 20 minutes

Ingredients
Serves 3–4

5 large heads bok choy

3 lbs shiitake mushrooms

3 shallots

1 tbsp sesame seeds

2 tbsps sesame oil

1 tbsp tamari, or to taste

Method

• Clean and pat dry bok choy and slice ends off. Set aside.

• Rinse mushrooms, pat dry, and slice thin.

• Peel shallots and slice thin.

• Bring one tablespoon sesame oil to medium heat in a skillet.

• Add shallots and cook for 3 minutes until caramelized.

• Add shiitake mushrooms and cook for 5 more minutes until golden brown and slightly crispy.

• Right before removing from pan, sprinkle in ½ tablespoon tamari and stir.

• Remove from pan and set aside.

• Add remaining tablespoon of sesame oil to skillet and bring to medium-high heat.

• Add bok choy and sauté 5 minutes until wilted and golden.

• In the last minute of cooking, add remaining ½ tablespoon soy sauce.

• Serve bok choy topped with shallots, shiitake mushrooms, and sesame seeds.

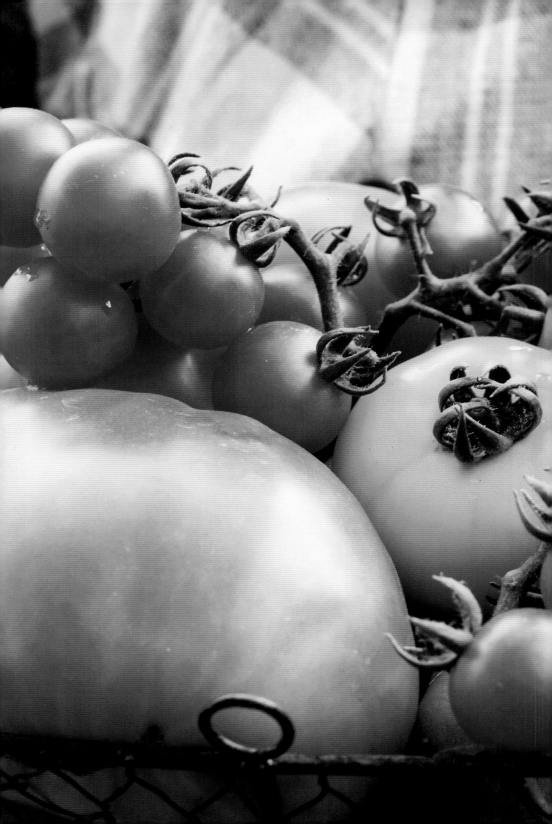

Summer Pasta Salad with White Beans, Tomatoes, and Basil Vinaigrette (V)

Prep time: 10 minutes
Cook time: 15 minutes

Ingredients
Serves 4–5

1 box favorite regular, whole wheat, brown rice, or gluten-free pasta

1 cup cooked white beans

2 cups diced tomatoes

2 bunches fresh basil

¼ cup olive oil

Sea salt, to taste

Black pepper, to taste

Method

• Cook your pasta of choice according to the box, strain, and transfer to large bowl.

• Add cooked white beans, diced tomatoes, sea salt, and pepper to taste.

• Blend basil with olive oil, sea salt, and black pepper to taste. If you need to thin the dressing, add more olive oil and/or water.

• Pour dressing over pasta, toss well, and serve with additional sliced fresh basil.

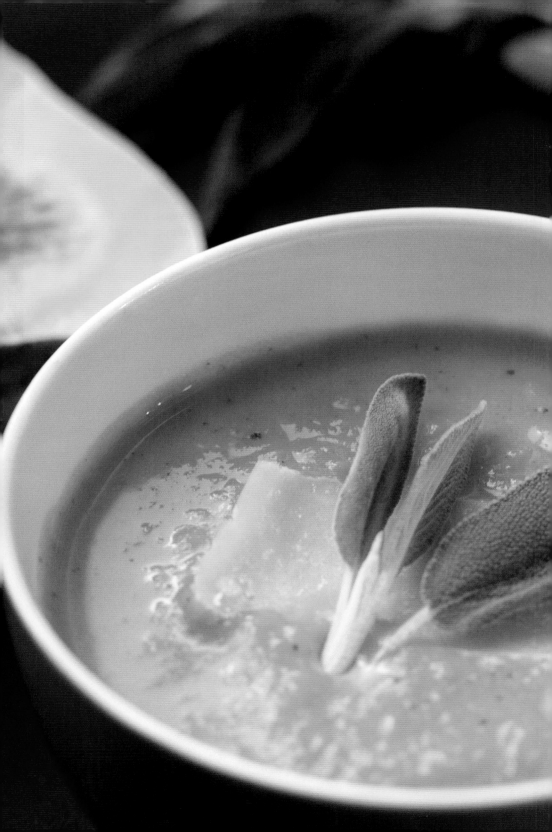

Butternut Squash Soup with Crispy Sage ⓥ ⒼⒻ

Prep time: 15 minutes
Cook time: 45 minutes

Ingredients
Serves 4–5

1 butternut squash

1 large yellow onion

3 stalks celery

3 carrots

3 cups vegetable stock

4 tbsps olive oil

¼ cup sage, sliced

Sea salt, to taste

Black pepper, to taste

Method

• Preheat oven to 350°F.

• Slice butternut squash in half (carefully!). Remove seeds and rub with olive oil, sea salt, and black pepper.

• Arrange skin-side up in large baking dish and cook for 30 minutes or until tender.

• While squash is cooking, rinse celery and carrots; peel carrots if not organic.

• Chop carrots and celery roughly. Peel onion and chop roughly.

• Add 3 tablespoons olive oil to large pot and bring to medium heat.

• Add onions and cook for 5 minutes.

• Add carrots and celery and cook for 8 more minutes.

• Add vegetable stock and bring to a boil; reduce heat, cover, and simmer until squash is done.

• Transfer roasted squash, vegetables, and broth to high-powered blender and combine until smooth.

• Add more salt and pepper if desired.

• Add one tablespoon olive oil to pan and bring to medium heat.

• Add sage and sauté until crispy.

• Serve soup with sage and black pepper.

IINsider Tip: Extra butternut squash? Make Roasted Mushrooms over Creamy Squash Purée ⓥ ⒼⒻ this week. (See page 145.)

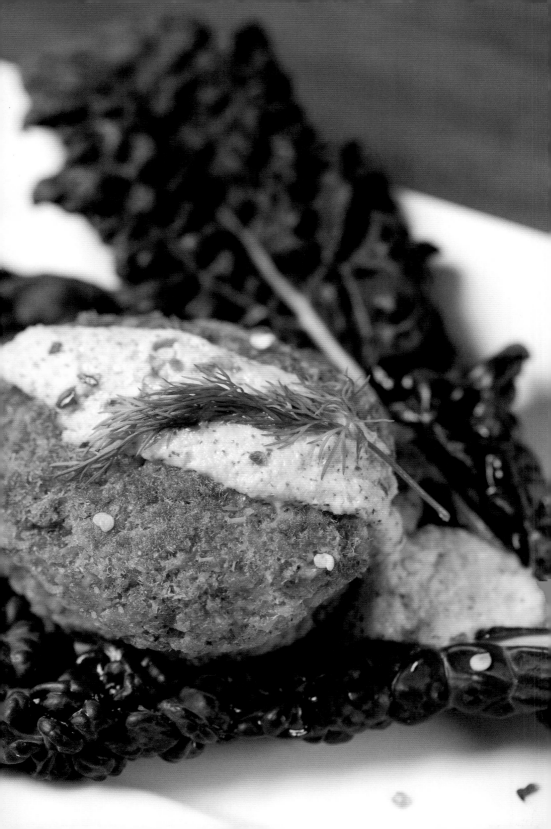

Salmon Burgers with Creamy Dill Sauce (DF)

Prep time: 4 hours
Cook time: 20 minutes

Ingredients
Serves 3–4

4–5 cans wild salmon (look for BPA-free) or 2 cups leftover grilled salmon, mashed

1 cup regular or gluten-free breadcrumbs

1 egg or egg substitute

1 cup cashews

Juice of 1 lemon

2 cloves garlic

1 bunch dill

¼ cup olive oil

¼ cup coconut milk

1 tbsp olive oil

½ cup chopped parsley

Sea salt, to taste

Black pepper, to taste

Method

• Soak cashews in water with a sprinkle of sea salt for 4 hours.

• Add salmon, breadcrumbs, parsley, sea salt, and pepper to large bowl and combine well using clean hands, or wear gloves.

• Once combined, beat egg in separate bowl and add to mixture. Combine well.

• Form mixture into small patties.

• Bring olive oil to medium-high heat in large skillet and cook burgers for 5 minutes on each side until cooked through and slightly crispy on the outside.

• For sauce, blend cashews, lemon juice, garlic, dill, olive oil, coconut milk, sea salt, and pepper on high speed until very creamy. Add more coconut milk and/or water if needed.

• Serve burgers on buns or over greens with sauce.

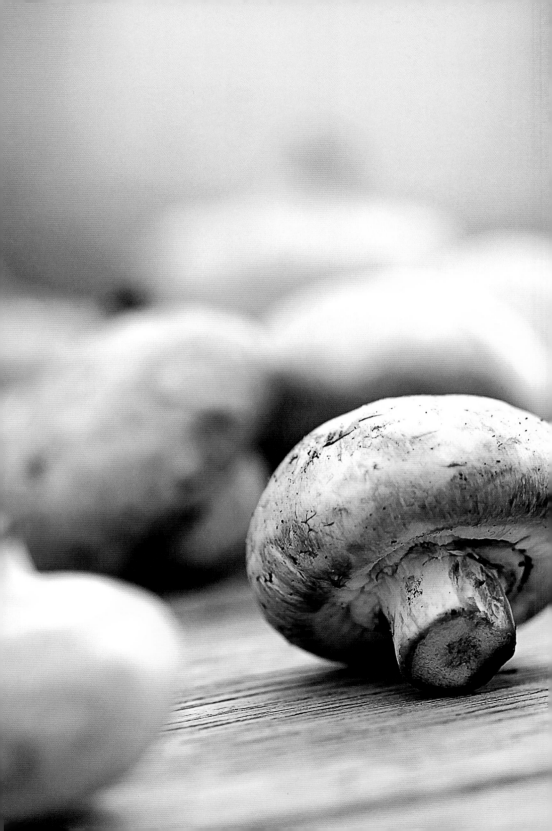

Lentil Mushroom Burgers (V) (GF)

Sarah Sunshine Kagan, Class of 2013

Prep time: 20 minutes
Cook time: 60 minutes

Ingredients
Serves 4

½ cup cooked brown rice

½ cup dry brown or green lentils

1 ½ cups chopped mushrooms of choice

1 shallot, diced

2 cloves garlic, minced

2 tbsps liquid amino acids

2 tbsps parsley, minced

1 tbsp flax seeds (optional)

1 cup water

1 tsp dried oregano

Olive oil

Method

- Preheat oven to 375°F.

- Line a baking sheet with tin foil and coat with cooking spray.

- Combine lentils and water in a pot.

- Bring to a boil, reduce, cover, and simmer for 20–30 minutes or until lentils are al dente.

- Cook shallot and garlic in one tablespoon olive oil, then add mushrooms and cook until they release most of their liquid.

- Add the lentils and liquid amino acids and cook until liquid is absorbed and the mixture starts to bind together (3–5 minutes).

- Remove from heat and add parsley, oregano, flax seed, and cooked brown rice.

- Use a masher to combine everything until thick paste forms.

- Divide into 4 patties of equal size.

- Bake for 25–30 minutes, flipping patties after 15 minutes.

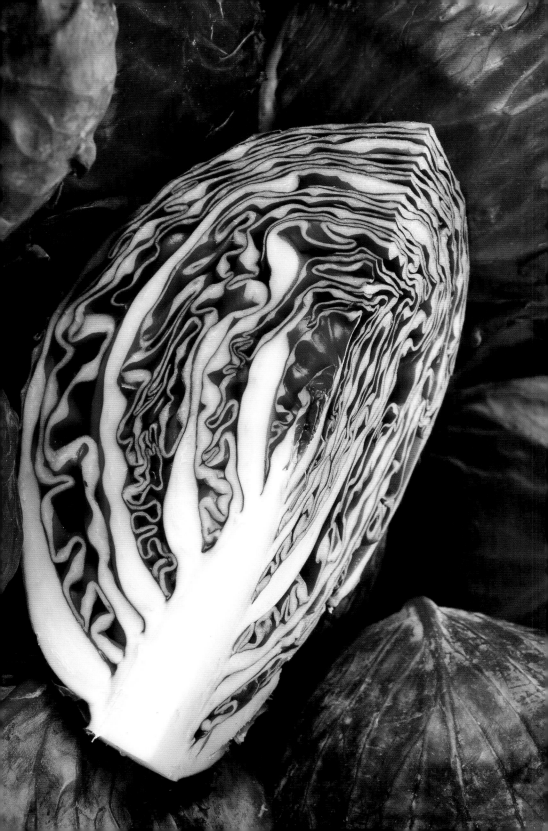

Chapter 7: Vegetarian

The vegetarian diet is a popular way to integrate more vegetables into your diet, be conscientious of the lives of animals, and eat more ethically. Even if you're not interested in giving up meat completely, you may want to try taking meat out of your diet one day a week. For example, Meatless Mondays are very popular. Experiment with the recipes in this chapter and notice how your body reacts.

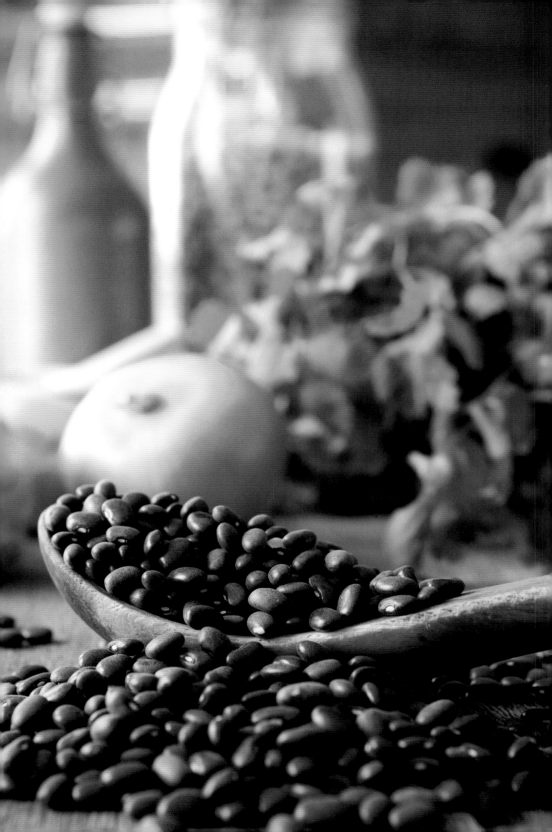

Black Bean Burgers

Prep time: 15 minutes
Cook time: 20 minutes

Ingredients
Serves 3–4

2 cups cooked black beans

¾ cup regular or gluten-free breadcrumbs

1 egg or egg substitute

1 medium yellow onion

1 tbsp cumin

1 tbsp chili powder, or to taste

2 tbsps olive oil

Sea salt, to taste

Black pepper, to taste

Method

- Bring one tablespoon olive oil to medium heat in medium pan.

- Peel and finely dice onion and add to pan. Cook for 5 minutes until caramelized.

- Combine black beans, breadcrumbs, cooked onion, cumin, chili powder, sea salt, and pepper in large bowl with clean hands. Massage mixture so black beans break down and form into dough.

- Beat your egg or egg substitute in separate bowl and add to main bowl, combining well.

- Form mixture into small-medium patties and cook in olive oil on medium-high heat in skillet for 5 minutes on each side, or until cooked through and slightly crispy on the outside.

- You can also grill these for a great smoky flavor.

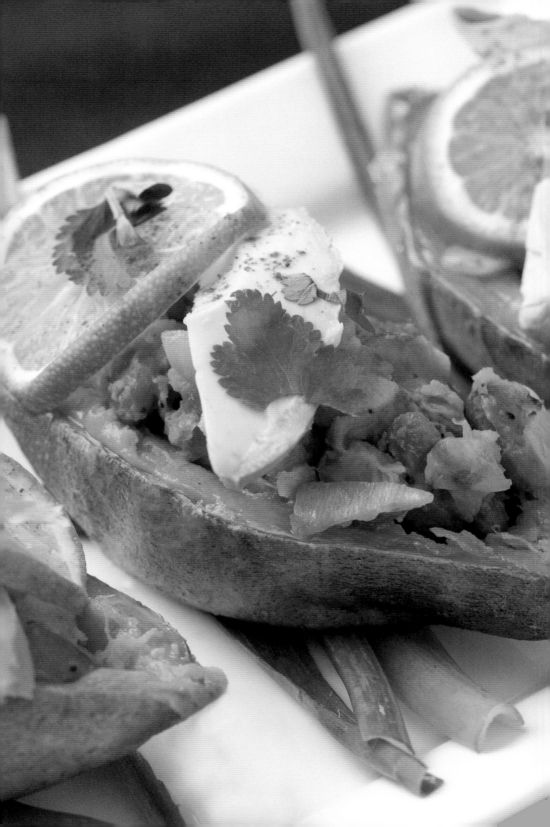

Stuffed Sweet Potatoes with Avocado, Black Beans, and Lime Vinaigrette Ⓥ ⒼⒻ

Prep time: 20 minutes
Cook time: 45 minutes

Ingredients

Serves 4

4 small-medium sweet potatoes

1 small yellow onion

1 cup cooked black beans

1 avocado

Juice of 5 limes

¼ cup olive oil and 1 tbsp olive oil

1 tbsp cumin

¼ cup chopped cilantro

Sea salt, to taste

Black pepper, to taste

Method

- Preheat oven to 350°F.

- Rinse sweet potatoes, pat dry, slice in half, and rub with one tablespoon olive oil.

- Lay on baking sheet and roast for 30 minutes or until fork tender.

- Remove from oven and scoop out most of the flesh, leaving a small amount so the skins keep their shape.

- While sweet potatoes are cooking, peel, dice, and sauté onion for 5–7 minutes in olive oil on medium heat in pan until caramelized.

- Transfer scooped out sweet potato flesh to pan with onion. Add cooked black beans, cumin, sea salt, and black pepper. Combine well.

- Stuff sweet potatoes with mixture.

- Transfer back to oven for 15 minutes.

- Whisk lime juice and ¼ cup olive oil with sea salt and black pepper to taste.

- Top stuffed sweet potatoes with diced avocado, cilantro, sea salt, black pepper, and lime vinaigrette.

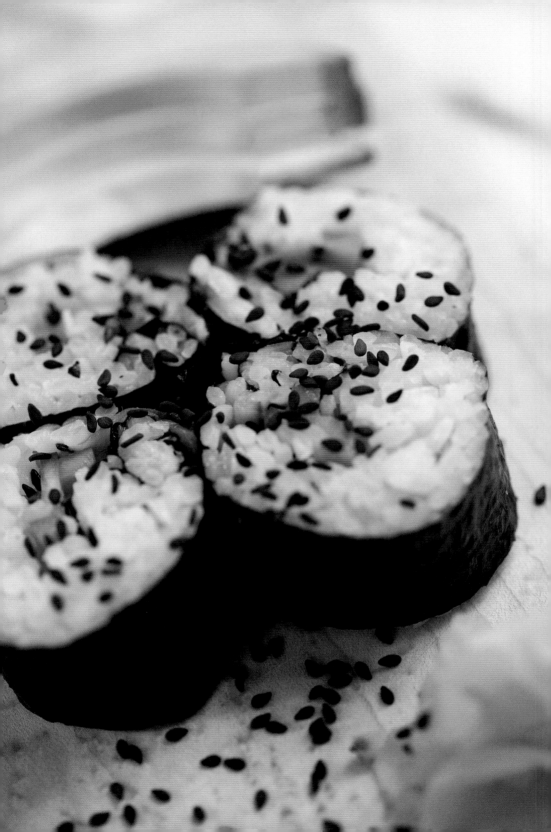

Carrot-Sesame Sushi with Avocado and Pickled Ginger Ⓥ ⒼⒻ

Prep time: 20 minutes
Cook time: 30 minutes

Ingredients
Serves 3–4

1 cup uncooked white sushi rice

1 ½ cups water

¼ cup coconut palm sugar

1 tbsp sesame oil

½ cup rice vinegar

1 tsp sea salt

1 avocado

4 sheets nori seaweed

2 carrots

3 tbsps sesame seeds

¼ cup good-quality pickled ginger (found at Japanese markets and health food stores)

Gluten-free tamari, for serving

Method

• Rinse uncooked rice in fine mesh strainer and transfer to medium pot.

• Add coconut palm sugar, sesame oil, rice vinegar, and sea salt.

• Bring to a boil, then reduce to lowest heat, cover, and cook for 20 minutes or until translucent and sticky.

• Lay one sheet of nori on top of sushi mat and press ½ cup rice into the center.

• Wash and slice carrots thin and lay them on top of rice.

• Add avocado slices.

• Add a thin layer of ginger (or to taste).

• Sprinkle with sesame seeds, then roll up tightly using the mat, remove the mat, and slice into 1-inch pieces.

• Repeat for all 4 sheets of nori.

• Serve with gluten-free tamari.

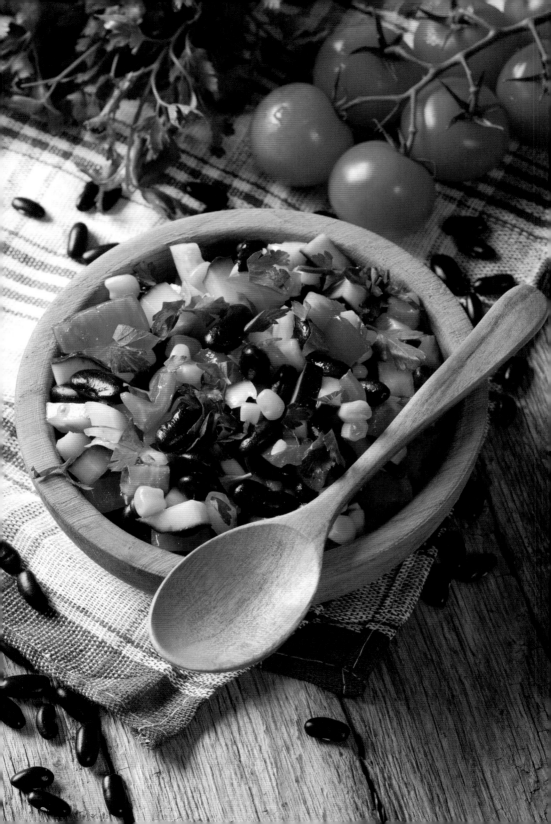

Hearty Mexican Bowl

Prep time: 15 minutes
Cook time: 0 minutes

Ingredients
Serves 1

¼ cup cooked corn

¼ cup cooked black beans

¼ cup Classic Quinoa (See recipe on p. 37)

¼ cup Peach Salsa (See recipe on p. 77)

1 cup Massaged Kale Salad (See recipe on p. 31)

2 tbsps Superfood Guacamole (See recipe on p. 73)

Juice of 2 limes

Sea salt, to taste

Black pepper, to taste

Method

• Toss corn and black beans with lime juice, sea salt, and black pepper to taste.

• Layer quinoa, then corn and black bean salad, then kale, peach salsa, and guacamole.

IINsider Tip: Leftover kale? Make Seared Steak with Super Green Chimichurri GF DF *this week. (See page 55.)*

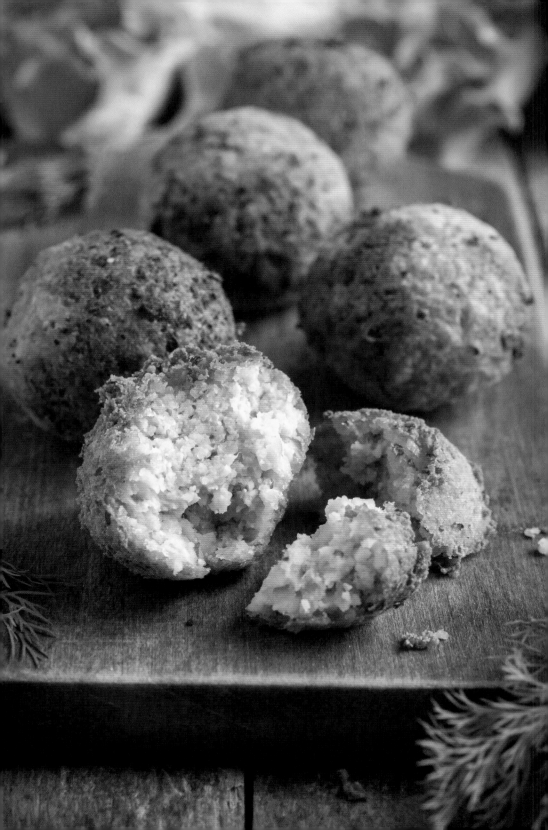

Falafels with Tzatziki

Prep time: 20 minutes
Cook time: 15 minutes

Ingredients
Serves 3–4

2 cups cooked chickpeas

⅓ cup regular or gluten-free flour

1 egg, beaten

1 medium yellow onion

3 cloves garlic

¼ cup fresh parsley

1 ½ tsps ground cumin

1 ½ tsps ground coriander

¾ tsp cayenne pepper, or to taste

1 cup Greek yogurt

1 English cucumber

1 tbsp minced fresh dill

1 tbsp apple cider vinegar

1 ½ tsps baking powder

Juice of 1 lemon

3 tbsps olive oil

4 tbsps safflower oil

Sea salt, to taste

Black pepper, to taste

Method

- Combine chickpeas, flour, beaten egg, parsley, cumin, coriander, cayenne, baking powder, sea salt, and black pepper in food processor until thick paste forms.

- Transfer to large bowl.

- Peel and dice onion and two cloves garlic and cook in two tablespoons olive oil for 5 minutes or until caramelized. Combine with chickpea mixture.

- Bring safflower oil to high heat in large skillet.

- Form chickpea mixture into 1-inch diameter balls and cook for 5 minutes on each side until cooked through and crispy.

For tzatziki

- Wash, pat dry, and grate cucumber.

- Mince one clove garlic and dill.

- Combine Greek yogurt, cucumber, garlic, dill, apple cider vinegar, lemon juice, one tablespoon olive oil, sea salt, and pepper in large bowl, mixing well.

Serve over falafels. Pair with your favorite Greek salad.

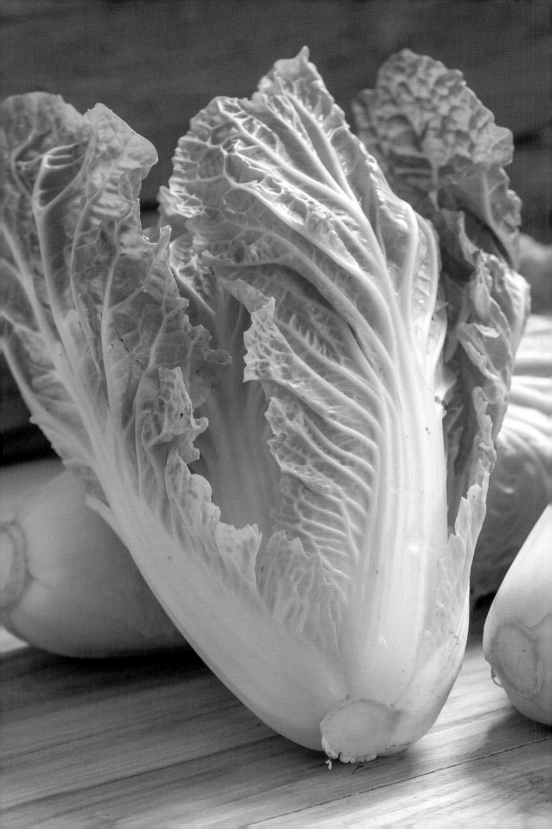

Pad Thai Salad

Dianne Wenz, Class of 2010

Prep time: 20 minutes
Cook time: 0 minutes

Ingredients

Serves 2–3

1 cup romaine lettuce, shredded

½ cup Napa cabbage, shredded

½ cup mung bean sprouts

1 red bell pepper, thinly sliced

2 carrots, shredded

1 package baked tofu, cubed

¼ cup chopped scallions

¼ cup chopped toasted peanuts

¼ cup lime juice

2 tbsps rice wine vinegar

2 tbsps tamari sauce

1 tbsp fresh grated ginger

1 tbsp natural creamy peanut butter

Hot chili sauce, to taste

Raw honey, to taste

Water, as needed

Method

- Blend lime juice, rice wine vinegar, tamari, ginger, peanut butter, chili sauce, honey, and water on high until well combined.

- Mix all salad ingredients together and divide between two plates or bowls.

- Top with dressing and garnish with scallions and peanuts.

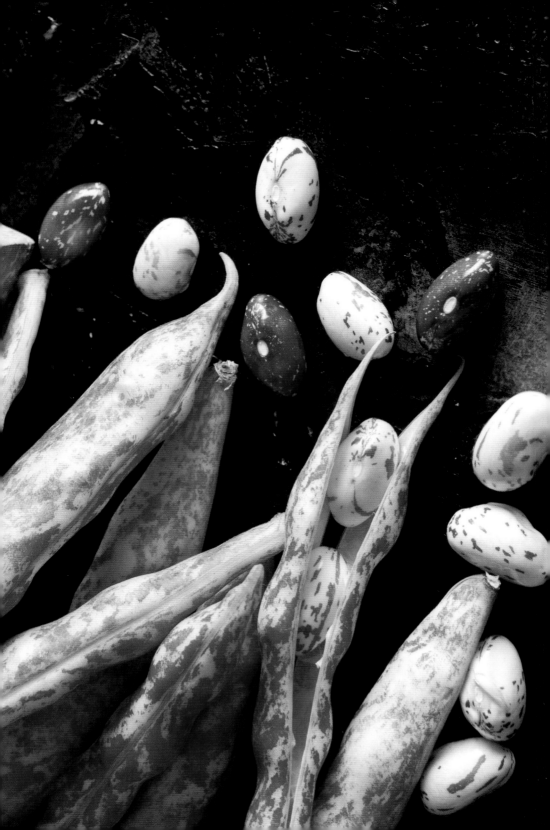

Chapter 8: Vegan

Vegans choose to avoid all animal products, including dairy, meat, eggs, and sometimes honey. For some people, a vegan diet greatly improves physical and emotional health by providing nutrients and eliminating toxins. It's also ethically sound since it honors animal rights and the survival of the planet. Even if going vegan doesn't work for you, try a few recipes from this chapter and experience how delicious animal-free food can be.

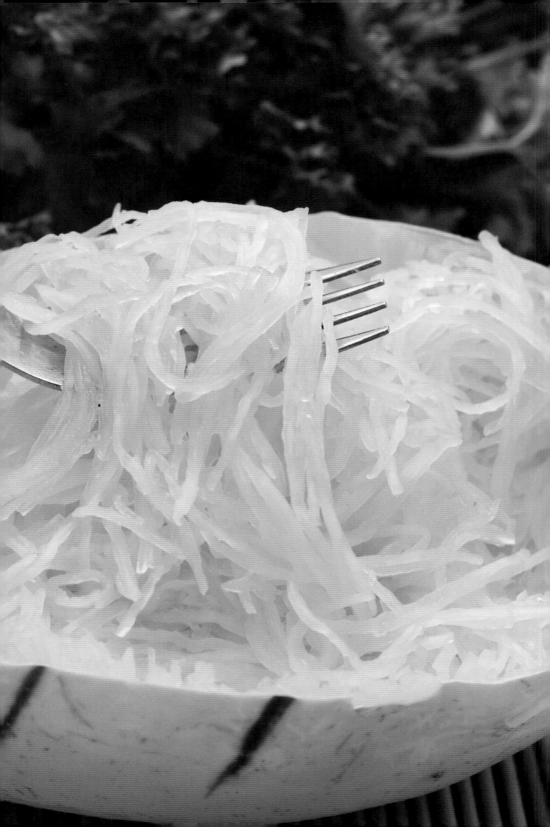

Spaghetti Squash with Caramelized Kale and Walnut Cream Sauce

Prep time: 4 hours
Cook time: 35 minutes

Ingredients
Serves 3–4

1 large spaghetti squash

1 cup walnuts

1 bunch lacinato kale

1 large yellow onion

½–1 cup vegetable stock

1 bunch fresh basil

5 tbsps olive oil

Sea salt, to taste

Black pepper, to taste

Method

• Soak walnuts in filtered water for 4 hours or overnight.

• Preheat oven to 350°F.

• Rinse, pat dry, and cut squash in half.

• Remove seeds and rub with olive oil, sea salt, and pepper.

• Lay skin-side up on baking dish and bake for 30 minutes or until fork tender.

• Scrape out "spaghetti" with spoon and set aside in bowl.

• Rinse and pat dry kale and remove leaves from stalks.

• Dice onion and caramelize in 2 tablespoons olive oil over medium heat for 5 minutes.

• Slice kale and add to pan. Allow to cook for 5 more minutes. Season with salt and pepper to taste.

• Transfer soaked walnuts, ½ cup vegetable stock, olive oil, sea salt, and black pepper to blender. Blend until smooth, adding more vegetable stock as needed.

• Layer caramelized onions and kale over spaghetti squash, then top with walnut cream sauce.

• Garnish with fresh basil and cracked black pepper.

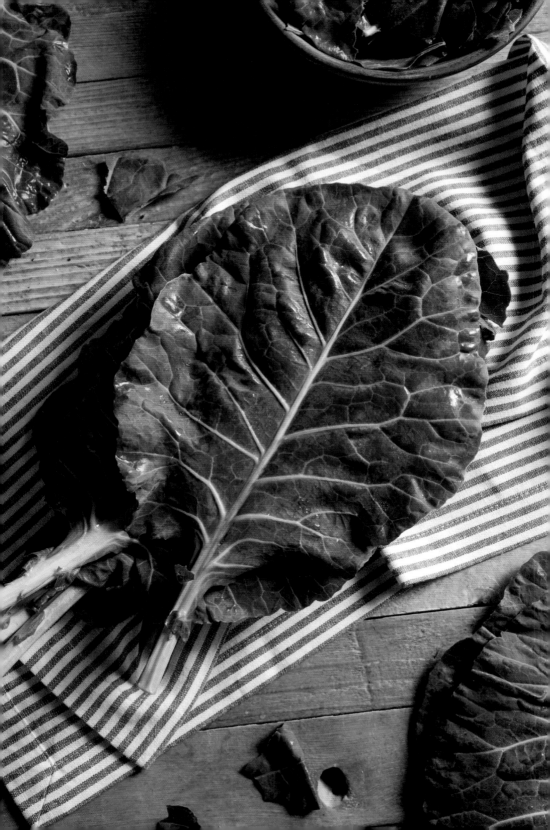

Grilled Tempeh Collard "Tacos"

Prep time: 15 minutes
Cook time: 50 minutes

Ingredients
Serves 4–5

2 packages tempeh of choice

5 large collard leaves

3 cups water

1 tbsp safflower oil

2 tbsps olive oil

2 tbsps cumin

1 tbsp chili powder

1 tbsp white pepper

1 tbsp black pepper

5–6 tbsps Superfood Guacamole (See recipe on p. 73.)

5–6 tbsps Peach Salsa (See recipe on p. 77.)

Sea salt, to taste

Black pepper, to taste

Method

• Bring salted water to a boil.

• Slice tempeh blocks into 4 pieces the short way. Add to boiling water and cook for 15 minutes. Strain and let cool.

• Combine cumin, chili powder, white pepper, black pepper, and sea salt in small bowl.

• Rub tempeh with mixture and set aside.

• Bring safflower oil to high heat in large grill pan, or use outdoor grill, and cook tempeh for 5 minutes on each side until golden brown.

• Remove, let cool for 5 minutes, and slice thin.

• Wash and pat dry collard leaves. Remove about half of the thick part of stalk. Cut collard leaves in half the long way.

• Toss with olive oil, sea salt, and pepper and allow to marinate for 5 minutes.

• Serve tempeh in collard leaf "tacos" with Superfood Guacamole and Peach Salsa.

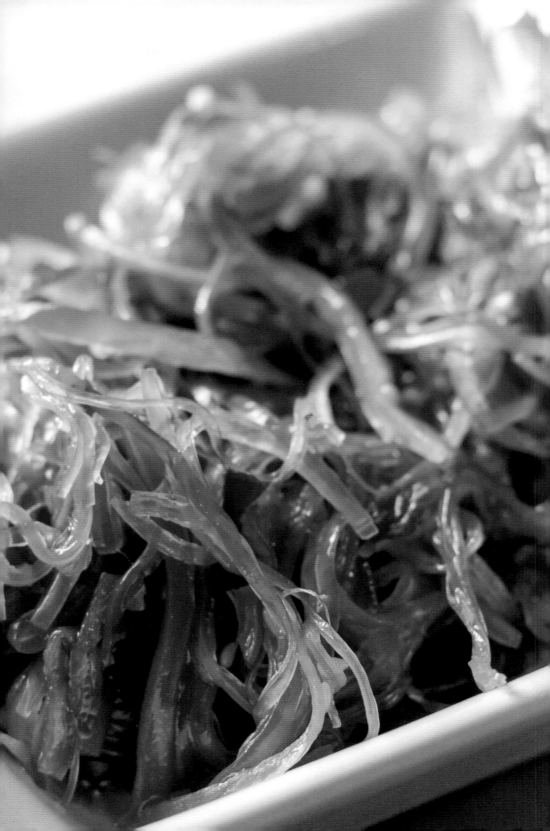

Seaweed and Fermented Vegetable Salad (V) (GF)

Prep time: 30 minutes
Cook time: 0 minutes

Ingredients
Serves 4–6

2 bunches collard greens

2 tbsps sesame oil

1 tbsp brown rice vinegar

2 cups cooked sushi rice

1 cup homemade pickled vegetables

4 cups water

½ cup hijiki or other seaweed (found at Japanese markets and health food stores)

2 tbsps sesame seeds

Method

- Rinse and pat dry collard greens. Remove from stock.

- Chop into small pieces and transfer to large bowl. Massage with sesame oil and brown rice vinegar for a minute.

- Soak dried hijiki in 4 cups of water for 30 minutes.

- Place ½ cup sushi rice in each bowl and top with collard greens, homemade pickled vegetables, and seaweed.

- Garnish with sesame seeds.

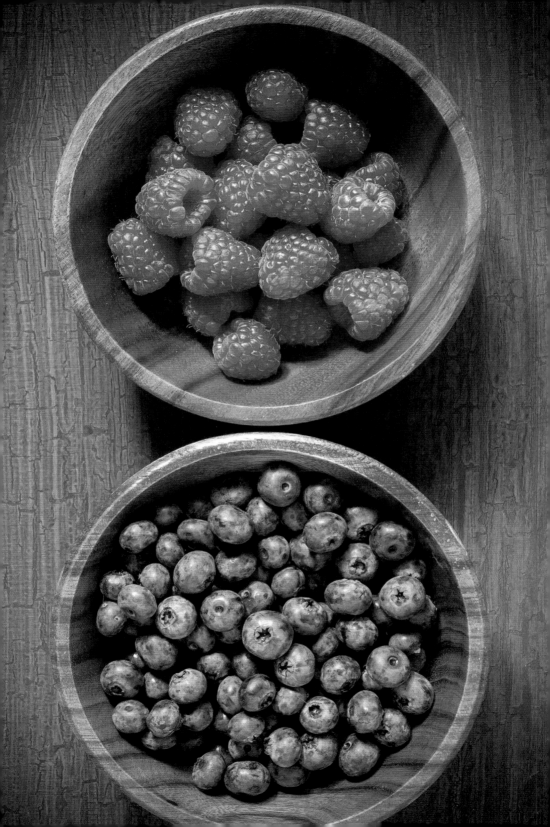

Sprout and Berry Salad with Zesty Lime Vinaigrette V GF

Prep time: 15 minutes
Cook time: 0 minutes

Ingredients
Serves 4–6

12 oz sprouts of choice

1 avocado

3 tbsps hemp seeds

1 cup blueberries

1 cup raspberries

¼ cup olive oil

Juice of 3 limes

Zest of 3 limes

Sea salt, to taste

Black pepper, to taste

Method

• Rinse and pat sprouts, blueberries, and raspberries dry.

• Add to large mixing bowl.

• Halve and score avocado into small cubes and add to bowl.

• Sprinkle with sea salt and black pepper.

• Add hemp seeds.

• In a separate bowl, whisk together olive oil, lime juice, lime zest, sea salt, and pepper.

• Pour over mixture and toss well.

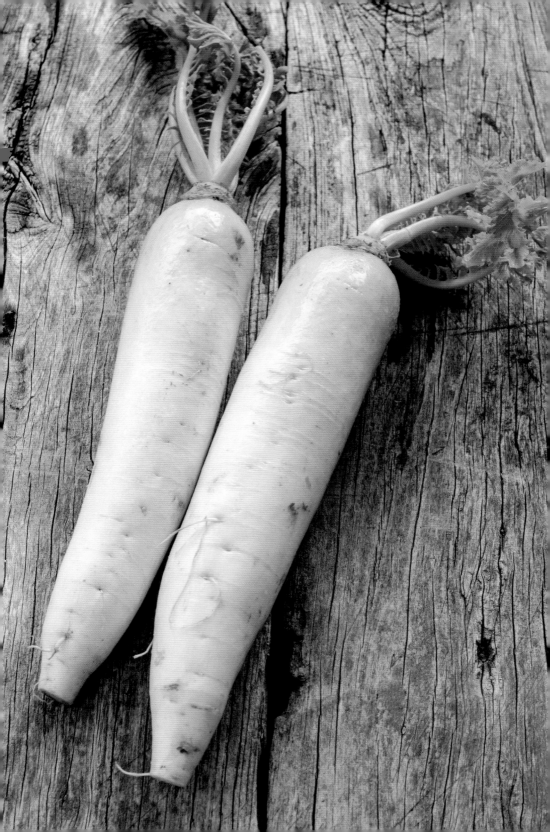

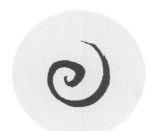

Grad Feature

Asian Abundance Bowl

Jade Kedrick, Class of 2014

Prep time: 30 minutes
Cook time: 0 minutes

Ingredients
Serves 1

3 leaves curly kale

1 cup arugula

2-inch daikon radish

½ cup hijiki

½ red bell pepper

½ avocado

2 tbsps sesame seeds

2 tbsps olive oil

1 tbsp sesame oil

2 tbsps umeboshi plum vinegar

2 ½ tbsps grated ginger (less if dried)

2 tbsps nutritional yeast

Method

- Soak hijiki for 20 minutes.

- Whisk together olive oil, sesame oil, umeboshi plum vinegar, ginger, and nutritional yeast to make your dressing.

- Add kale to large bowl and massage in half the dressing until kale is tender.

- Add arugula, daikon radish, hijiki, bell pepper, avocado, and sesame seeds to large mixing bowl.

- Toss well with rest of dressing and serve.

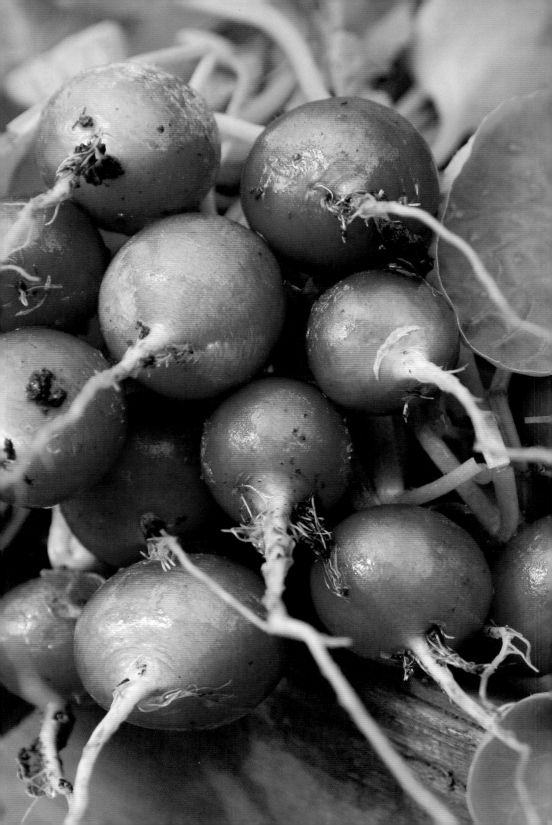

Chapter 9: Grain-Free

Removing grains from your diet may help lower insulin levels, reduce internal inflammation, and improve digestion. Followers of the grain-free approach believe that grains are not necessary for optimal health. Grain-free does not translate to taste-free—the grain-free recipes in this chapter will boost your energy, nurture your soul, and keep your taste buds happy.

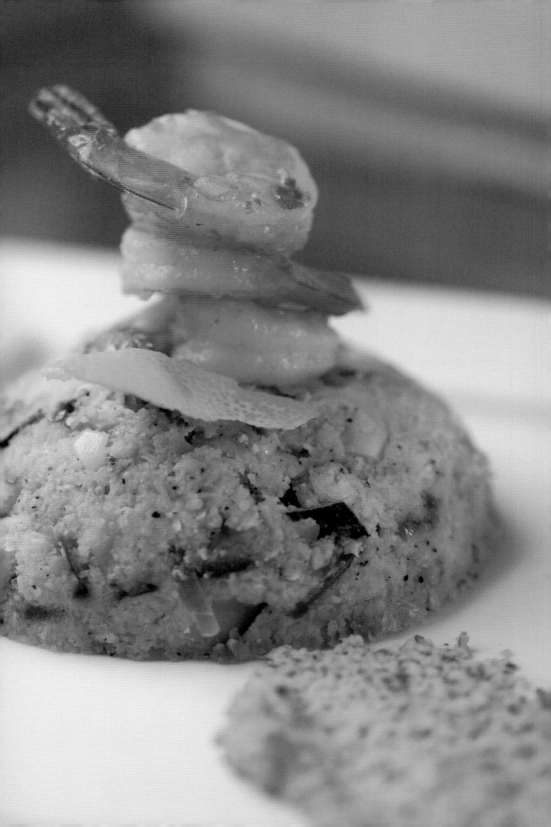

Cauliflower Rice with Grilled Shrimp and Spicy Drizzle

Prep time: 25 minutes
Cook time: 10 minutes

Ingredients
Serves 3–4

1 head cauliflower

1 medium yellow onion

2 cloves garlic

1 large zucchini

¾ lb large shrimp

1 cup almonds

½ cup water

2 tbsps favorite hot sauce, or to taste

2 tbsps olive oil

Juice of 1 lemon

Sea salt, to taste

Black pepper, to taste

Method

• Wash cauliflower and pat dry. Trim ends and transfer to food processor. Pulse until "rice" forms. Set aside in large bowl.

• Peel and dice onion and garlic and add to pan with olive oil on medium heat. Cook for 5 minutes or until caramelized.

• Wash, pat dry, and dice zucchini and add to pan. Cook for 5 more minutes.

• Transfer vegetable mixture to cauliflower and toss well. Add lemon juice and olive oil. Add salt and pepper to taste.

• Peel, devein, rinse, and pat shrimp dry.

• Bring olive oil to medium-high heat in pan and cook shrimp for 3 minutes on each side until cooked through and opaque. Add salt and pepper to taste. Set aside.

• Add almonds, ½ cup water, favorite hot sauce, sea salt, and pepper to blender or food processor and blend on high until creamy sauce forms. Add more water if needed.

• Serve shrimp over "rice" with spicy drizzle.

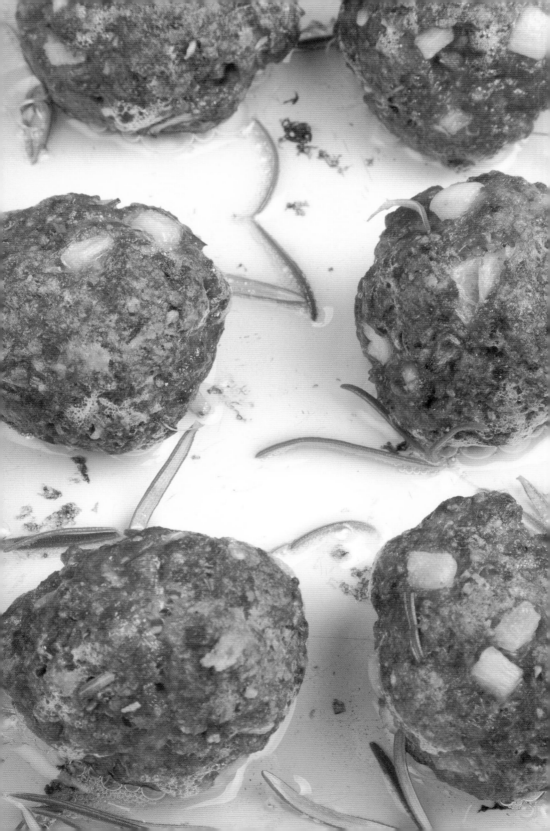

Favorite Rosemary Meatballs

Prep time: 15 minutes
Cook time: 25 minutes

Ingredients
Serves 4–5

½ lb ground beef, grass-fed, organic and/or local

½ lb ground pork, grass-fed, organic and/or local

½ cup almond meal

1 egg

1 medium yellow onion

3 sprigs rosemary

4 tbsps olive oil

Parsley, to garnish

Chili flakes, to taste

Sea salt, to taste

Black pepper, to taste

Method

- Bring 2 tablespoons olive oil to medium-high heat, dice onion, and cook for 5 minutes or until caramelized.

- Chop rosemary and add to pan and stir. Add salt and pepper to taste.

- Transfer ground beef and pork, almond meal, salt, and pepper to large mixing bowl.

- Add caramelized onion-rosemary mixture to main bowl.

- Beat egg in separate bowl and add in. Combine all ingredients well.

- Bring 2 tablespoons olive oil to medium-high heat in large skillet and cook meatballs for 7 minutes on each side until golden brown and cooked through completely.

- Serve meatballs with your favorite vegetable and garnish with parsley and chili flakes if desired.

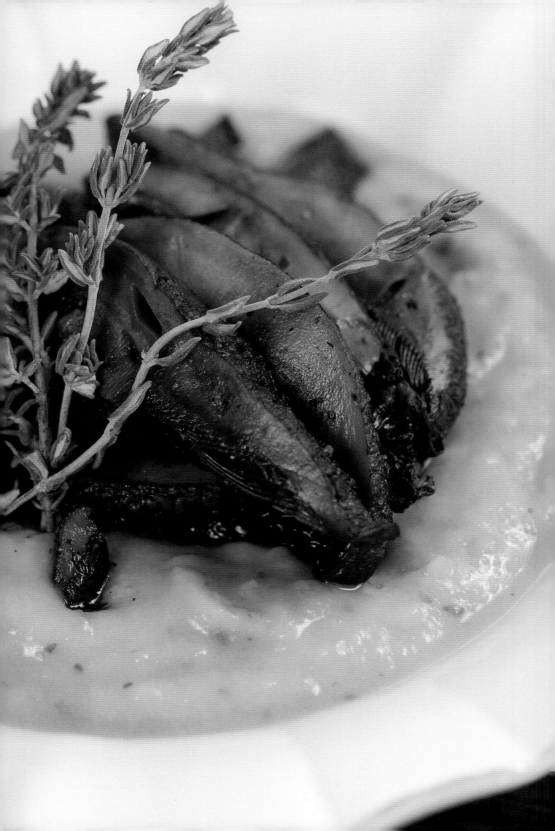

Roasted Mushrooms over Creamy Squash Purée

Prep time: 15 minutes
Cook time: 50 minutes

Ingredients
Serves 3–4

4–5 portobello mushroom caps

1 butternut squash

½–1 cup pure coconut milk

4 tbsps olive oil

2 tbsps dried thyme

Sea salt, to taste

Black pepper, to taste

Method

- Preheat oven to 350°F.

- Rinse squash, pat dry, cut in half, de-seed, and rub outside with olive oil, salt, and pepper.

- Place skin-side up on baking sheet and transfer to oven. Cook for 30 minutes or until tender.

- Rinse and pat portobello caps dry.

- Rub with olive oil, thyme, salt, and black pepper and transfer to baking dish.

- Roast for 15 minutes at 350°F until cooked through.

- When squash is done, remove from oven and cool.

- Peel, dice, and add to food processor along with coconut milk, sea salt, and pepper.

- Blend until thick and creamy. Use more coconut milk if needed.

- Serve roasted mushrooms over squash purée and garnish with thyme sprig.

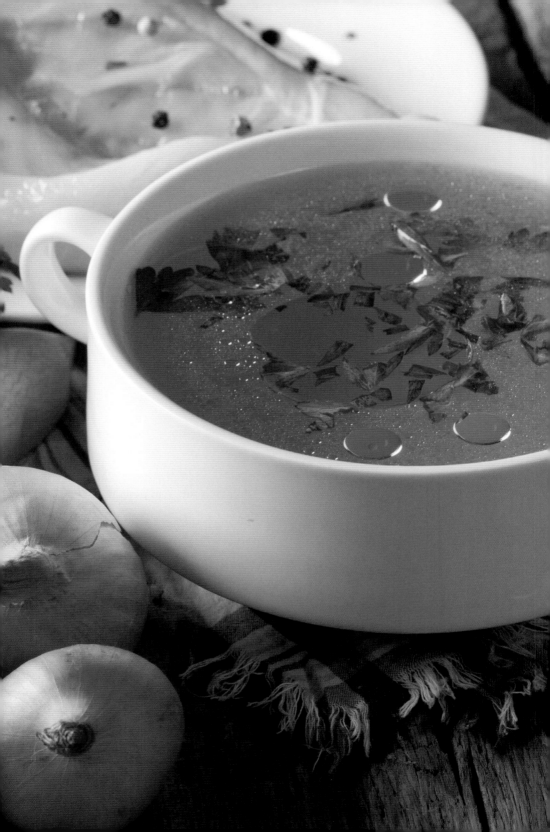

Chicken and Vegetable Soup

Prep time: 15 minutes
Cook time: 90 minutes

Ingredients
Serve 6–8

3–4 cooked chicken breasts, local, and/or organic

1 large yellow onion

3 stalks celery

3 large carrots

5 cups chicken stock (organic, homemade, or boxed)

¼ cup minced rosemary

3 tbsps olive oil

Sea salt, to taste

Black pepper, to taste

Method

• Peel and dice onion.

• Wash and pat celery dry and chop onions, carrots, and celery into small cubes.

• Bring olive oil to medium heat in large pot and add onion. Cook for 5 minutes until caramelized.

• Add celery and carrots and cook for 7 more minutes.

• Sprinkle with sea salt and pepper.

• Add rosemary and combine well.

• Add chicken stock and bring to boil.

• Reduce heat and simmer for one hour.

• Shred or cube chicken and add.

• Cook for 10–15 more minutes and serve.

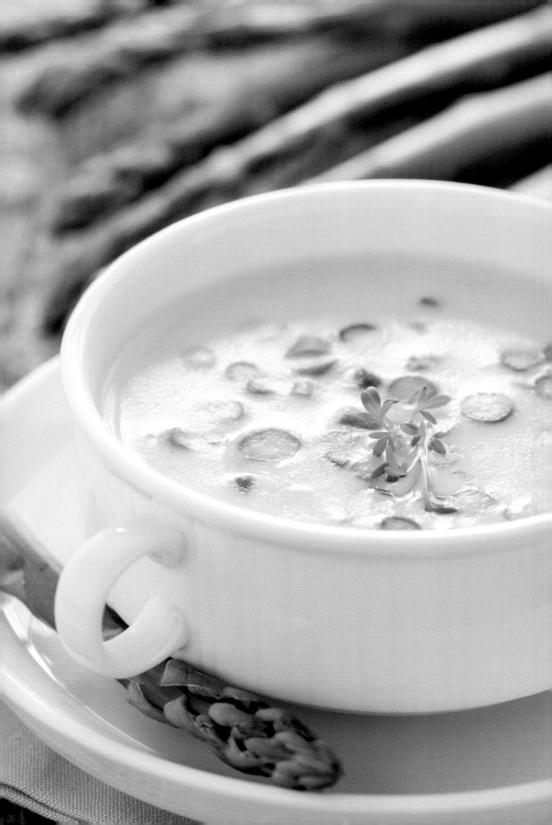

Creamy Asparagus Soup

Prep time: 15 minutes
Cook time: 50 minutes

Ingredients
Serves 4–5

2 bunches asparagus

1 large yellow onion

5 stalks celery

3 cups vegetable stock
(organic, homemade,
and/or boxed)

¼ cup minced thyme

3 tbsps olive oil

Sea salt, to taste

Black pepper, to taste

Method

• Peel and dice onion.

• Wash celery and asparagus and pat dry, then
  chop into ¼-inch pieces.

• Bring olive oil to medium heat in large pot
  and add onion.

• Cook for 5 minutes until caramelized.

• Add celery and asparagus and cook for
  7 more minutes.

• Sprinkle with salt and pepper.

• Add thyme and combine well.

• Add vegetable stock and bring to boil.

• Reduce heat and simmer for 30 minutes.

• Transfer to blender or food processor and
  blend on high until creamy.

• Garnish with thyme.

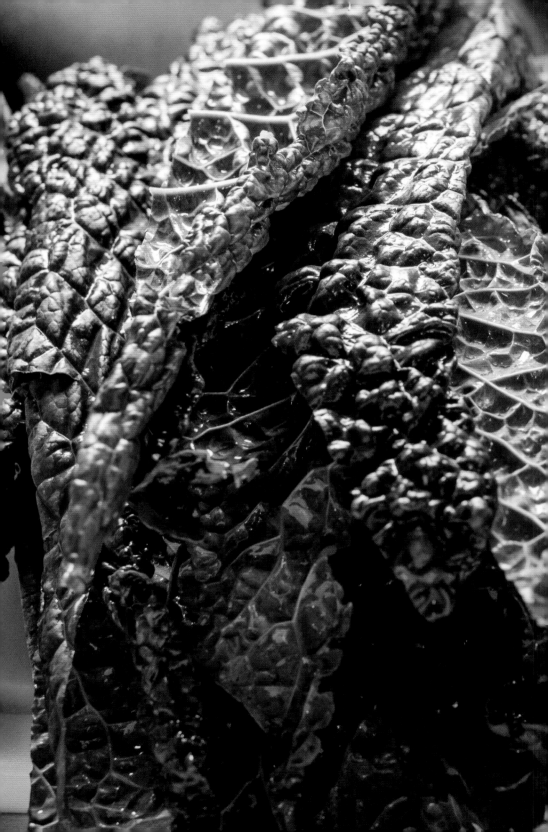

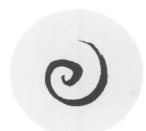

Grad Feature

Massaged Kale with Fried Egg VG GF

Rachel Shulman, Class of 2012

Prep time: 15 minutes
Cook time: 10 minutes

Ingredients
Serves 4

1 bunch kale

Juice of ½ lemon

¼ cup raw almonds

½ cup cherry tomatoes

¼ cup extra virgin
olive oil

4 medium eggs

2 tbsps butter or
coconut oil

¼ tsp ground cumin

Sea salt, to taste

Black pepper, to taste

Grated pecorino
cheese (optional)

Method

• Wash and pat kale dry and slice into ribbons.

• Combine in large bowl with olive oil and lemon juice. Massage until kale softens.

• Toast almonds in a skillet over medium heat until lightly browned.

• Remove almonds from heat and, once cooled, finely chop.

• Cut cherry tomatoes in half.

• Add almonds and tomatoes to kale and mix well.

• Add cumin and season with salt and pepper.

• In a skillet, fry eggs in butter or coconut oil.

• Top salad with fried eggs and shaved pecorino cheese, if desired.

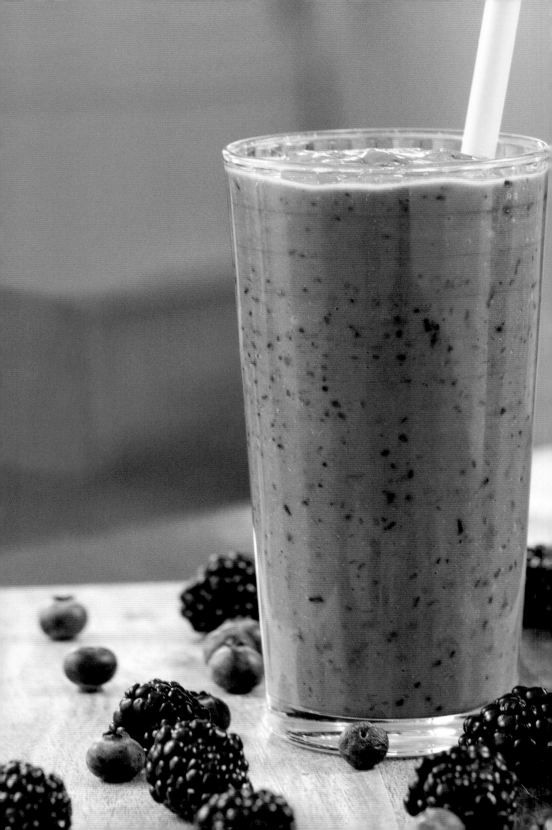

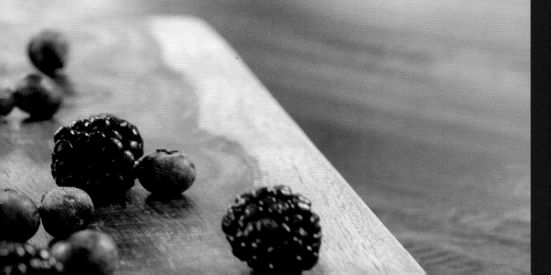

Raise a Glass to Health

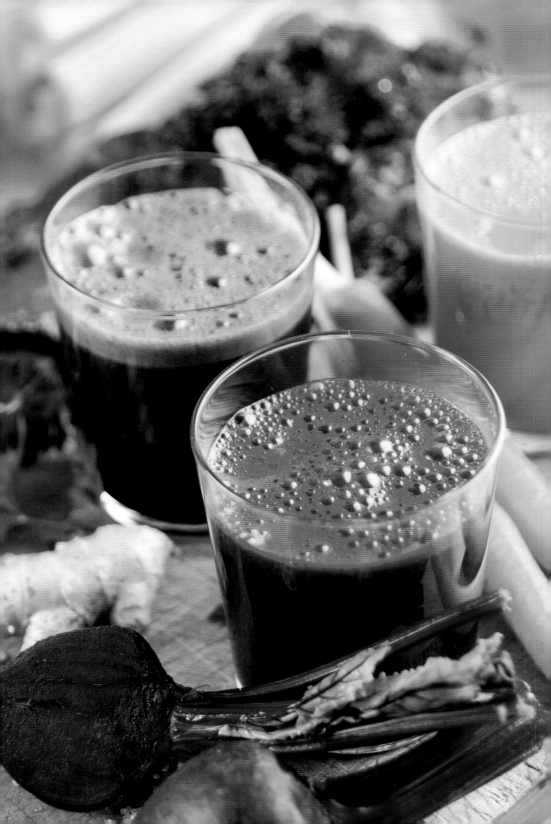

Chapter 10: Juices

The Juices chapter is one of my absolute favorites. Green juice in the morning, a juice right after a hard workout, a juice just when you want a juice—juices are everywhere. I love juicing and dropped 20 pounds doing it. If you don't have a juicer, you can even blend your produce and then strain it through a nut milk bag. Here are a few easy and nutritious combinations to get you started.

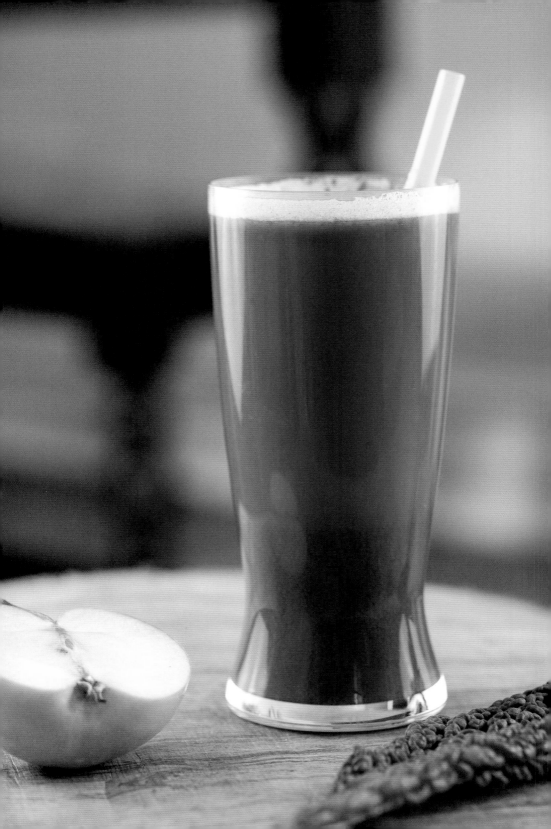

Pure Sunshine Green Juice

Prep time: 10 minutes
Cook time: 0 minutes

Ingredients

Serves 2

5 leaves kale

2 large English
cucumbers

2 green apples

1 lemon

Options

¼ cup fresh basil
or mint

⅛ cup coconut milk

Method

• Rinse all ingredients and peel if they aren't
organic.

• Slice cucumbers the long way, so you have
spears.

• Core apple.

• Cut lemon into four.

• Pass all ingredients through juicer.

• Option: Blend juice with ⅛ cup coconut milk
for a creamier version.

Pro Tip: *If you don't have a juicer, don't worry. Simply follow the steps above,
but instead of passing everything through a juicer, combine well in a blender then
pass through a nut milk bag.*

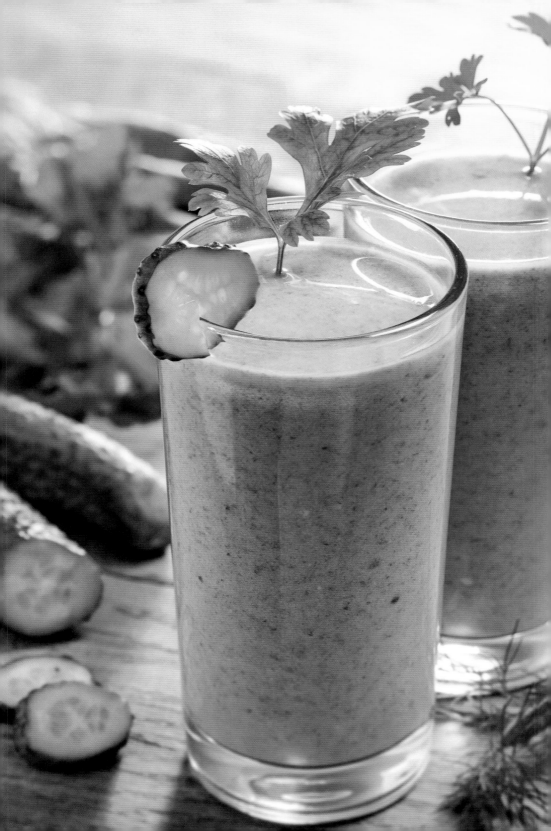

Super Greens

Prep time: 10 minutes
Cook time: 0 minutes

Ingredients
Serves 2

5 leaves Swiss chard

2 large English
cucumbers

5 stalks celery

1 cup loose-packed
parsley

1 lemon

1-inch ginger, or less,
to taste

Method

• Rinse all ingredients and peel if they aren't
  organic.

• Slice cucumbers the long way, so you have
  spears.

• Trim celery ends.

• Cut lemon into four.

• Pass all ingredients through juicer.

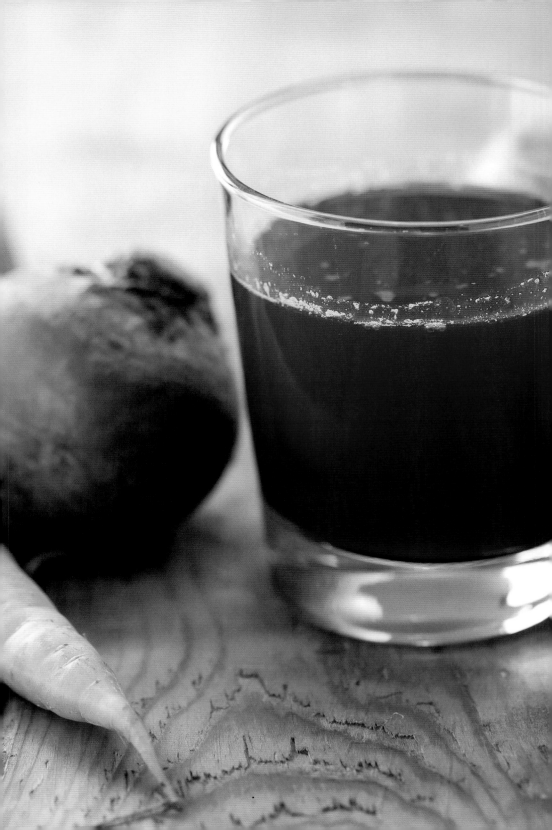

Rooted

Prep time: 10 minutes
Cook time: 0 minutes

Ingredients
Serves 2

7 large carrots

5 large beets

4 large green apples

1 lemon

1-inch piece ginger

Method

• Rinse all ingredients and peel if they aren't organic.

• Trim carrot and beet ends.

• Core apple.

• Cut lemon into four.

• Pass all ingredients through juicer.

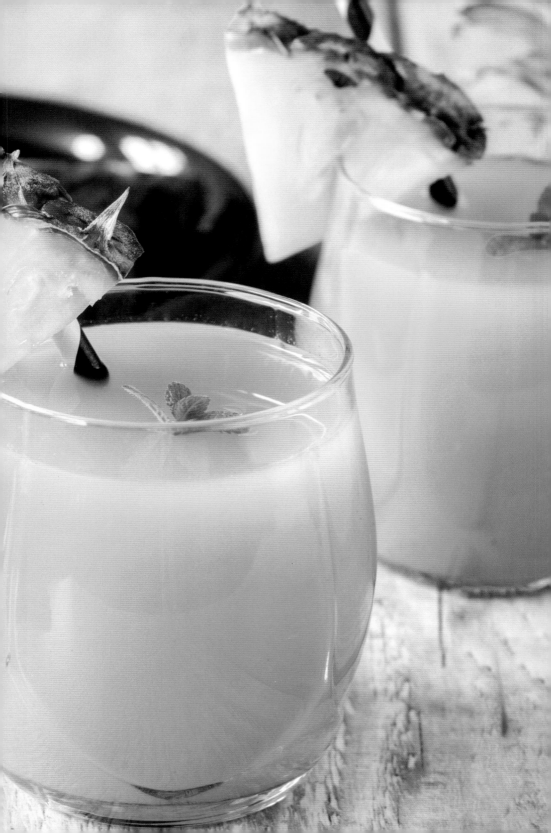

Pineapple-Lemon Zinger

Prep time: 10 minutes
Cook time: 0 minutes

Ingredients
Serves 2

1 pineapple

2 large English cucumbers

1 green apple

1 lemon

Method

• Rinse all ingredients and peel if they aren't organic.

• Core pineapple and chop.

• Slice cucumbers the long way, so you have spears.

• Core apple.

• Cut lemon into four.

• Pass all ingredients through juicer.

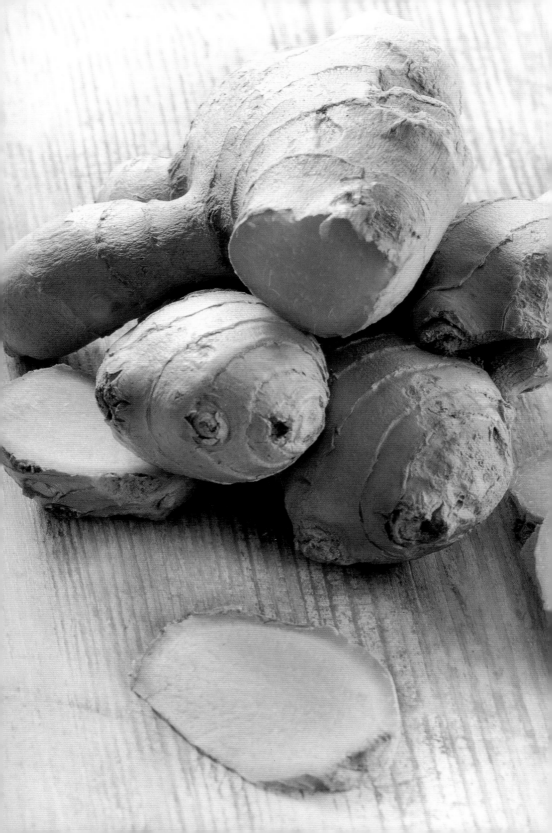

Cold Cure

Prep time: 10 minutes
Cook time: 5 minutes

Ingredients
Serves 2

7 green apples

2-inch piece ginger

1 tsp cayenne pepper,
or less, to taste

1 tsp cinnamon

Method

• Rinse all ingredients and peel if they aren't organic.

• Core apples and chop into fours.

• Pass apples and ginger through juicer.

• Transfer to pot along with cayenne and cinnamon.

• Warm on medium-low heat and enjoy.

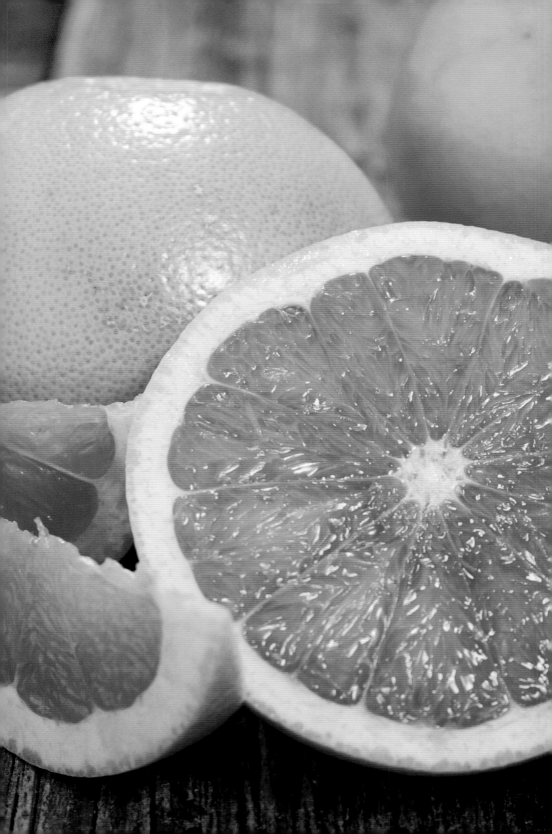

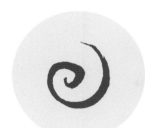

Playful Juice

Aubrey Levitt, Class of 2015

Prep time: 10 minutes
Cook time: 0 minutes

Ingredients
Serves 1

1 grapefruit

1 green apple

½ cucumber

Handful of spinach

Pinch of dill

Method

• Rinse all ingredients and peel if they aren't organic.

• Cut grapefruit and apple into fours.

• Slice cucumber into spears.

• Juice all ingredients.

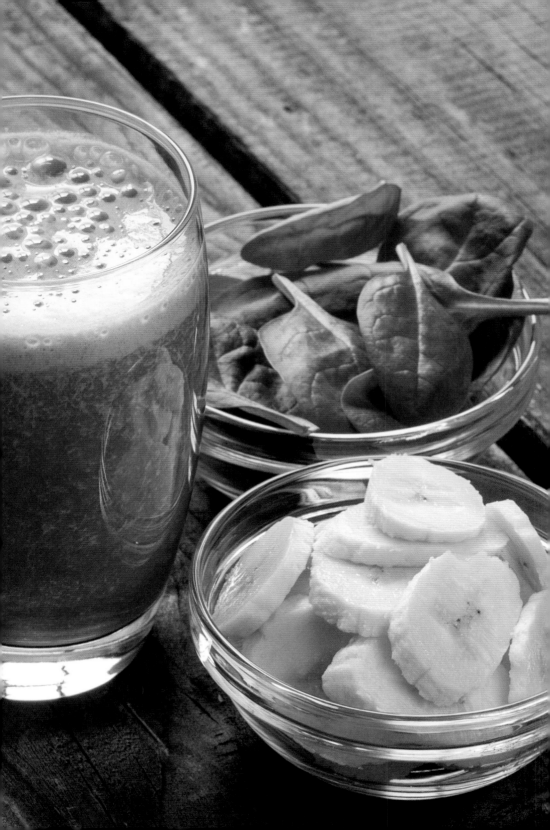

Chapter 11: Smoothies

Smoothies are a quick and easy way to get a lot of nutrients into your body. Whether you're on the go or just in the mood to sip your breakfast slowly on a relaxing morning, smoothies can ensure that your body is nourished throughout the day. They are also a great way to sneak in extra vegetables, the most common missing food group in the modern diet. This chapter is great for busy people who want to maximize their nutrient intake.

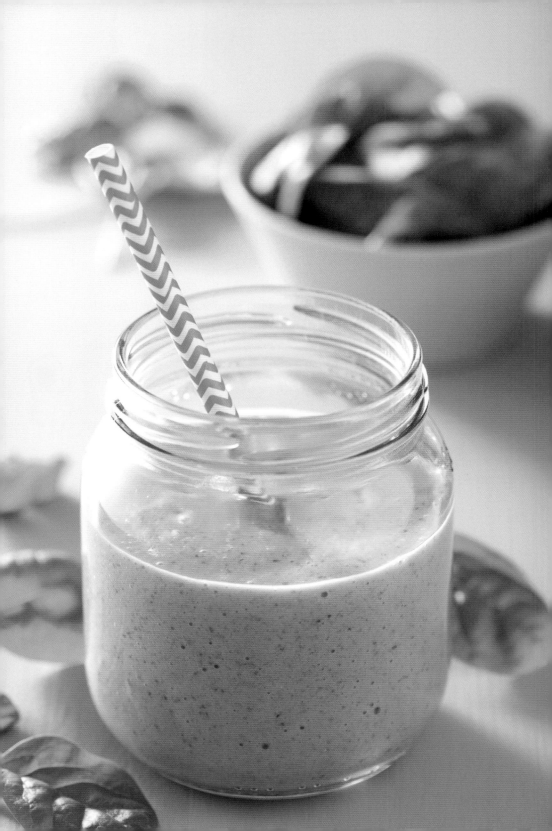

Green Smoothie

Prep time: 5 minutes
Blend time: 5 minutes

Ingredients
Serves 2

2 loose-packed cups kale or spinach

2 frozen bananas (freeze overnight)

1 green apple

1 cup almond milk

Method

• Freeze peeled bananas in chunks to have on hand.

• Wash greens and apples.

• Core apples and cut into fours.

• Transfer all ingredients to blender and blend on high until creamy, adding more almond milk if needed.

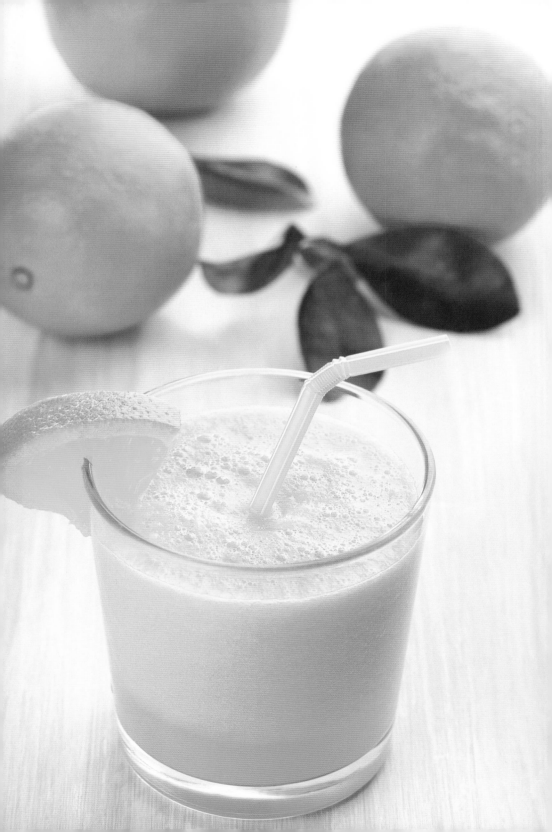

Citrus Smoothie

Prep time: 5 minutes
Blend time: 5 minutes

Ingredients
Serves 2

2 frozen bananas
(freeze overnight)

1 small English
cucumber

2 oranges

1 cup coconut milk

Juice of 1 lemon

Method

• Freeze peeled bananas in chunks to have
  on hand.

• Wash all ingredients and peel if not organic.

• Cut lemon in half.

• Roughly chop oranges.

• Transfer all ingredients to blender and blend
  on high until creamy, adding more coconut
  milk if needed.

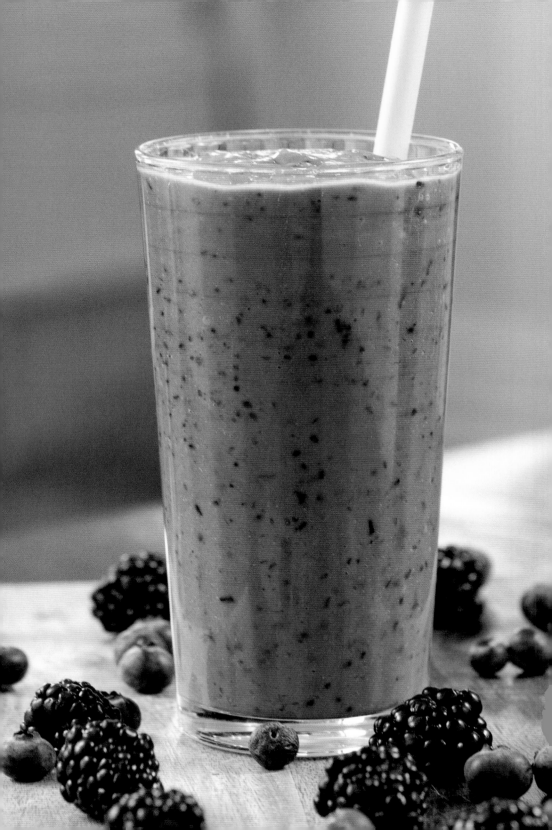

Creamy Berry Smoothie

Prep time: 10 minutes
Blend time: 5 minutes

Ingredients
Serves 2

1 avocado

1 cup blueberries

1 cup blackberries

2 tbsps chia seeds

Juice of 2 limes

1 cup almond milk

5 ice cubes

Method

• Wash and pat all produce dry.

• De-pit and score avocado and transfer to blender.

• Add remaining ingredients and blend on high until smooth and creamy.

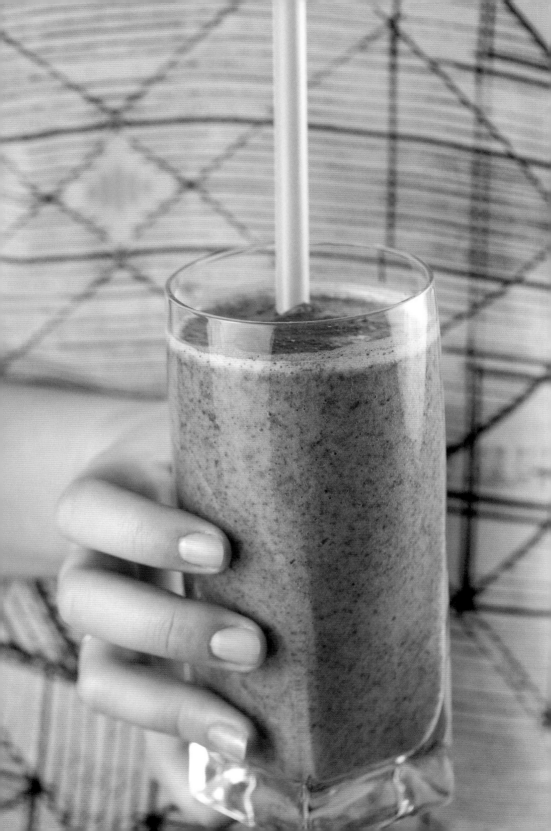

Superfood Cacao Smoothie

Prep time: 5 minutes
Blend time: 5 minutes

Ingredients

Serves 2

2 frozen bananas
(freeze overnight)

2 tbsps maca

1 tsp cinnamon

2 tbsps raw cacao

2–3 pitted dates, or to taste

1 cup cashew milk or milk of choice

Method

- Freeze peeled bananas in chunks to have on hand.

- Blend all ingredients until creamy, adding more cashew milk if needed.

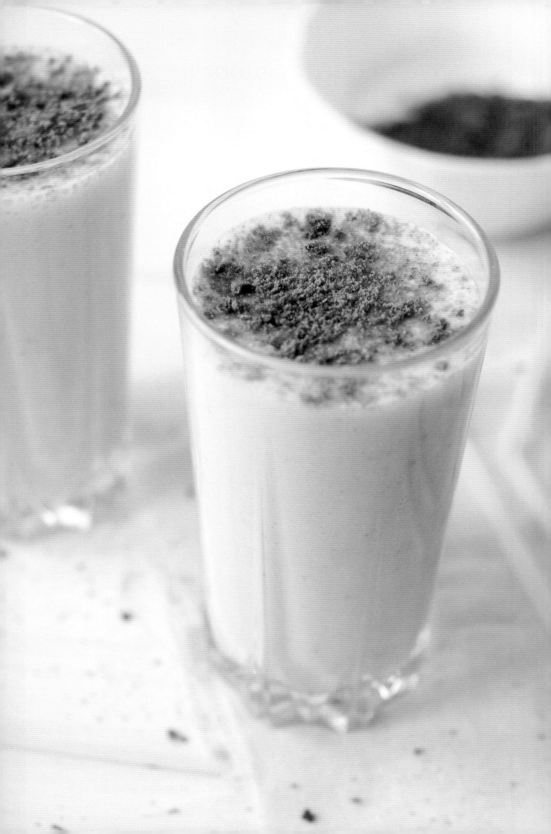

Creamy "Horchata" Smoothie

Prep time: 5 minutes
Blend time: 5 minutes

Ingredients
Serves 2

2 frozen bananas
(freeze overnight)

2 tbsps sesame seeds

½ cup cooked gluten-
free oatmeal

1 tbsp cinnamon

2–3 pitted dates, to taste

1 cup rice milk or
other milk of choice

5 ice cubes

Method

• Freeze peeled bananas in chunks to have
on hand.

• Blend all ingredients until smooth and
creamy, adding more milk if needed.

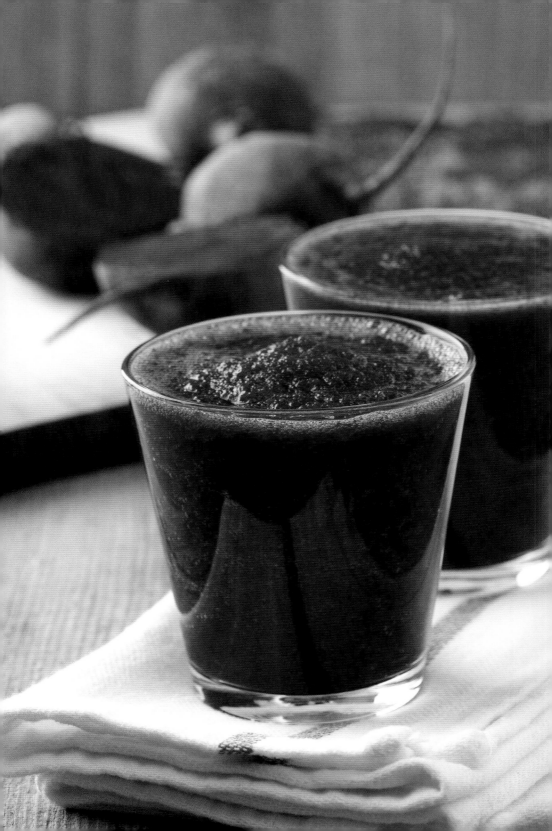

Red Beet, Carrot, and Apple Smoothie GF

Sarah Sunshine Kagan, Class of 2013

Prep time: 10 minutes
Blend time: 10 minutes

Ingredients
Serves 2–3

1 sweet apple

½ cup cooked and peeled beets

1 cup carrots, softened

1 cup almond milk, milk of choice, or water

1½ tsps fresh ginger, minced

1 tbsp flaxseed

5 ice cubes

Method

• Bring one cup water to a boil and add the carrots. Boil 3–5 minutes until soft. Allow to cool.

• Cut apple into chunks and add everything to the blender.

• Whirl away and enjoy!

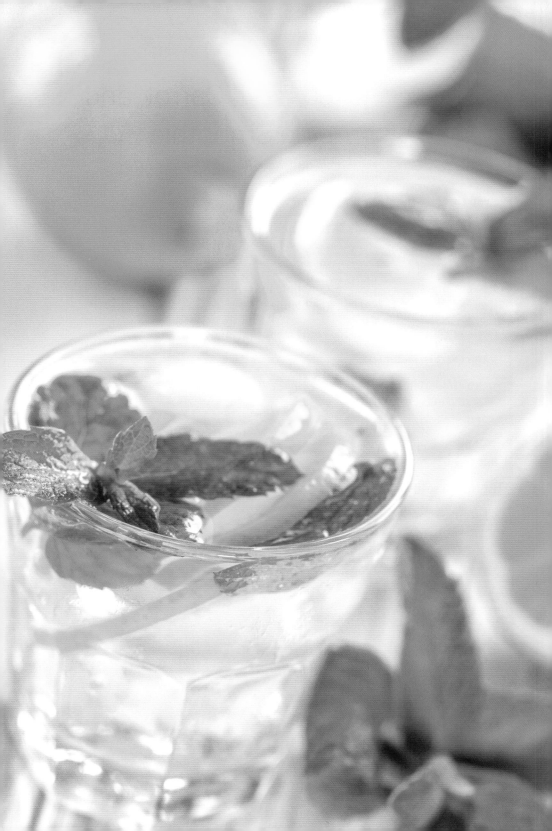

Chapter 12: Healthy Beverages

Staying hydrated is crucial to staying healthy. Liquids help with stagnation and other digestive issues, keeping the mind sharp, and controlling appetite. Often when you're hungry, you really just need a glass of water or two. In this chapter, you'll find beverages that will hydrate your system, rev up your metabolism, and boost your immunity. Next time you're hungry, try one of the drinks from this chapter first.

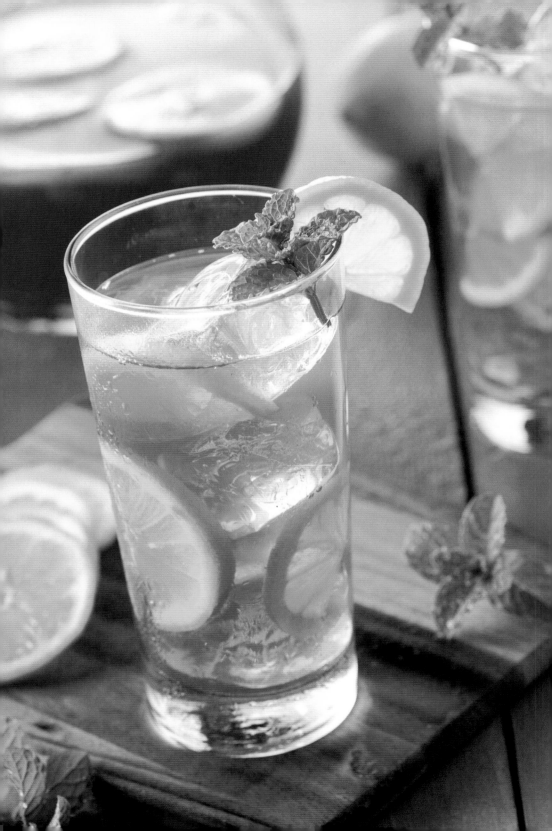

Iced Mint Tea with Lemon and Honey (V) (GF)

Prep time: 10 minutes
Cook time: 5 minutes

Ingredients

Serves 2

3 cups strong brewed mint tea

Juice of 1 lemon

1 tbsp honey (optional)

Method

• Dissolve honey in warm mint tea and add lemon juice.

• Pour into pitcher filled with ice and serve.

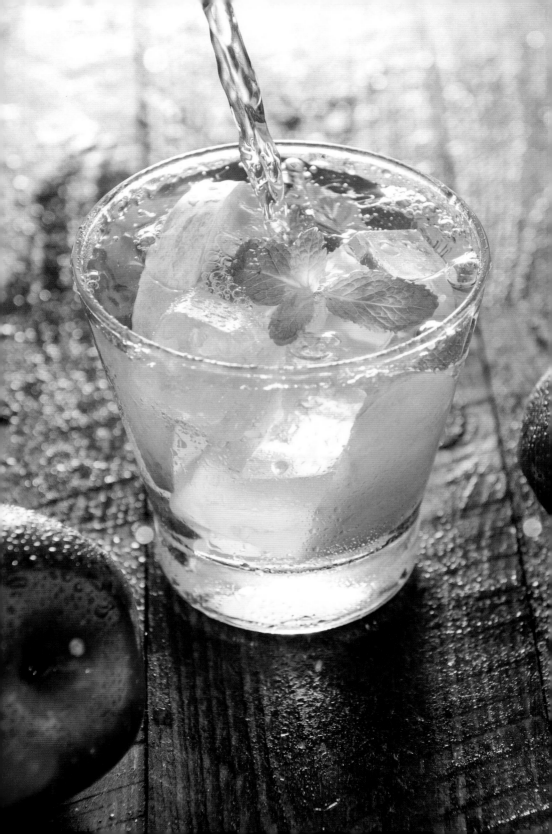

Iced Kukicha with Apple and Lemon (V) (GF)

Prep time: 10 minutes
Cook time: 5 minutes

Ingredients
Serves 2

3 cups strong brewed kukicha tea (found at health food stores, often called bancha or twig tea)

½ cup fresh apple juice

Juice of 1 lemon

Method

• Wash apple and lemon and peel if not organic.

• Core apple, chop lemon in half, and pass both through juicer.

• Combine with brewed kukicha, pour over ice, and serve.

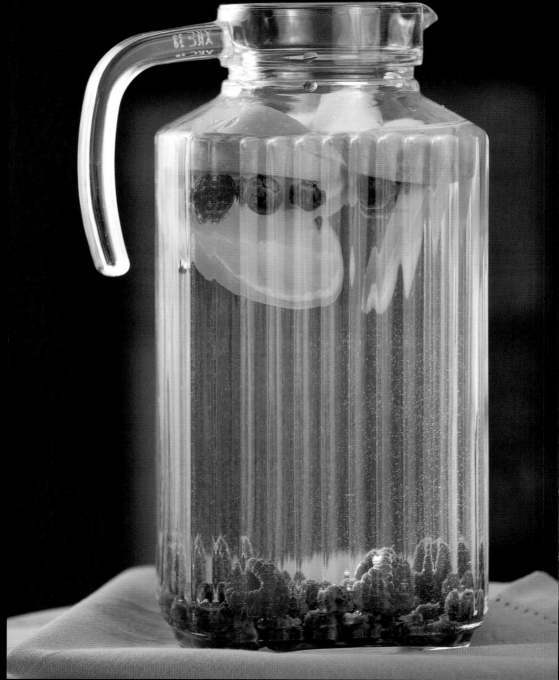

Basic Fruit Water

Prep time: 10 minutes
Cook time: 0 minutes

Ingredients
Serves 2

2 quarts water

1 cup blueberries

1 cup raspberries

1 green apple

2 limes

Method

- Wash all fruit.

- Peel apple if not organic, core, and chop.

- Chop lime.

- Add all fruit to pitcher with ice and fill with filtered water.

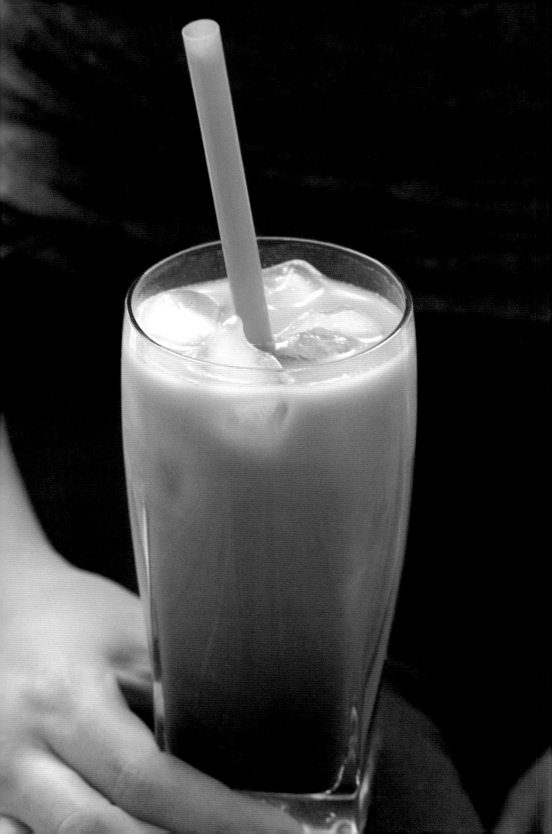

Cold Brew Coffee

Prep time: 8 hours
Cook time: 0 minutes

Ingredients
Serves 3–4

⅓ cup freshly ground, organic, medium roast coffee

1 cup filtered, room temperature water

Options

Sweetener of choice

Milk of choice

Mint leaves

Coconut oil

Vanilla bean or extract

Cinnamon

Cardamom

Method

Concentrate:
• Combine freshly ground coffee and water in glass mason jar with lid.

• Stir well with a wooden spoon or chopstick. Avoid metal utensils since it changes the flavor. The grinds will float to the top.

• Seal jar and let sit overnight (at least 8 hours) on countertop or in fridge, depending on your temperature preference.

• Pour mixture through a fine mesh strainer into another jar to remove grinds. Your concentrate will stay fresh for up to one week.

• Dilute ¼ cup concentrate with ¾ cup water and add your favorite milk and/or sweetener.

• You may also warm the coffee on a stovetop for hot coffee, which will still be far less acidic than traditionally brewed coffee.

Options

• For stronger coffee, add more grounds at the beginning.

• Add two sprigs of fresh mint to your soaking jar for a great herbal flavor.

• Blend brewed coffee with one teaspoon coconut oil, ¼ cup coconut milk, and ½ vanilla bean or one teaspoon vanilla extract for a delicious frothy beverage.

• Add cinnamon or cardamom.

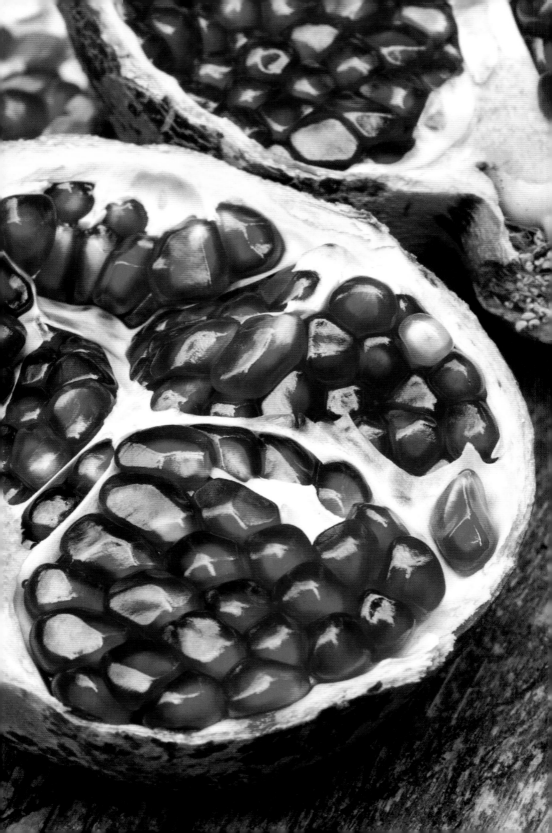

Classic Sangria

Prep time: 15 minutes
Cook time: 0 minutes

Ingredients
Serves 4

2 bottles favorite
red wine

¾ cup orange juice

½ cup brandy

¼ cup triple sec

¾ cup blueberry or
pomegranate juice

½ cup honey simple
syrup

1 green apple

1 orange

Method

• Combine red wine, orange juice, brandy,
triple sec, and blueberry or pomegranate
juice in large pitcher and stir well.

• Dissolve ¼ cup honey in warm water and stir
into pitcher.

• Wash apple and orange, core apple, cut all
into thin slices, and add to pitcher.

• Serve.

• Option: Omit the alcohol (red wine, brandy,
and triple sec) and use kombucha for a
fun, sparkling, non-alcoholic, gut-friendly
alternative. You may also want to omit the
honey simple syrup since kombucha is sweet.

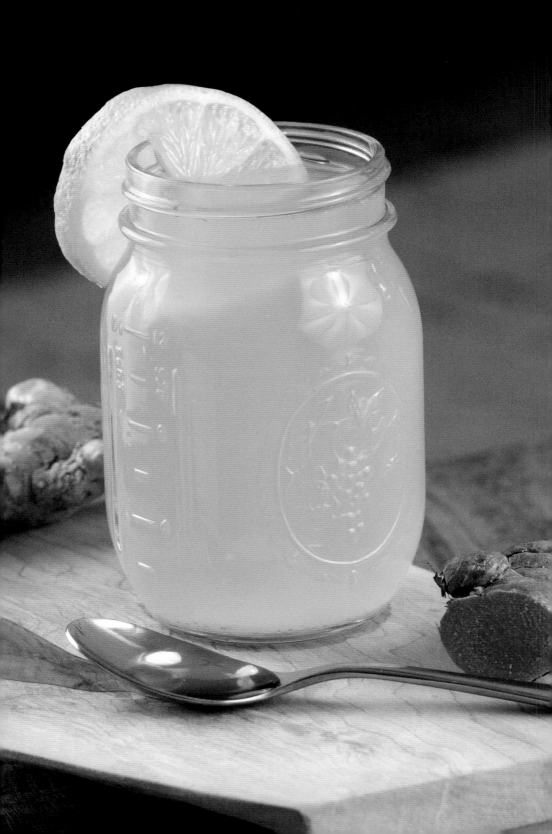

Warming Ginger-Turmeric Tea

Prep time: 10 minutes
Cook time: 5 minutes

Ingredients
Serves 2

3 cups brewed fresh or bagged ginger tea

1 tsp turmeric

Juice of 1 lemon

1 tbsp honey (optional)

Method

- Brew tea and mix in turmeric, lemon juice, and honey.

- Stir well and serve.

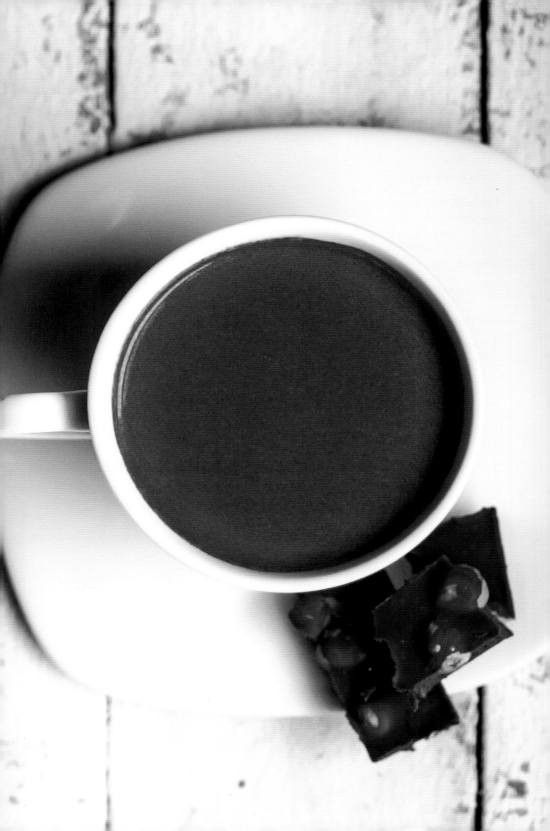

Grad Feature

Healthy Homemade Hot Chocolate

Andrea Hood, Class of 2013

Prep time: 5 minutes
Cook time: 5 minutes

Ingredients
Serves 1–2

1 can coconut milk

2 tbsps raw cacao powder (or unsweetened cocoa powder)

2 tbsps pumpkin puree

2 tbsps pure maple syrup

¼ tsp pumpkin pie spice

Method

• Blend all ingredients until combined and smooth for about 30 seconds.

• Pour into a saucepan and warm over medium heat, stirring occasionally for approximately 5 minutes.

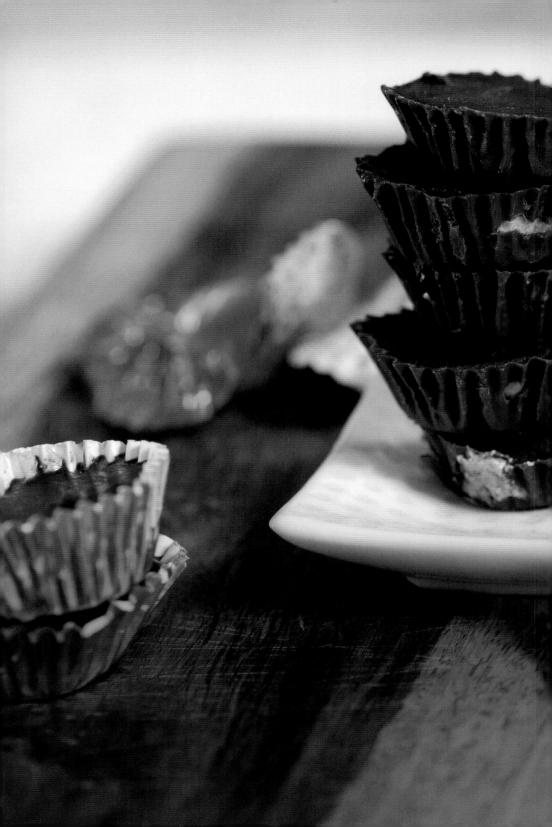

Superfood Sweets

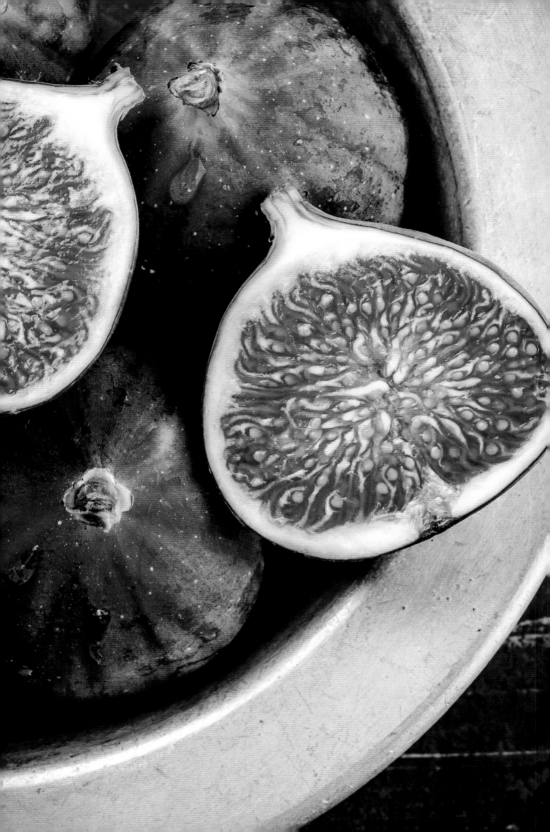

Chapter 13: Superfood Sweets

A lot of people have a sweet tooth, and that's okay. By eating sweet vegetables to crowd out sugar cravings, you can naturally reduce—not necessarily remove—sweets from your diet. It's all about what you *can* eat, not what you *can't* eat. In this section, I've chosen some of my favorite superfood desserts that are packed with flavor and won't weigh you down. Keep in mind that these are still treats, so eat sparingly.

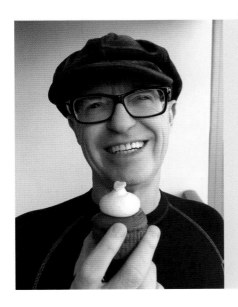

"In any relationship, if one partner is loving, faithful, and supportive, it's easy for the other to take that person for granted. That's what most of us do with our bodies. It is time for you to shift this, and working to understand your cravings is one of the best places to begin. Then you can build a mutually loving relationship with your own body."

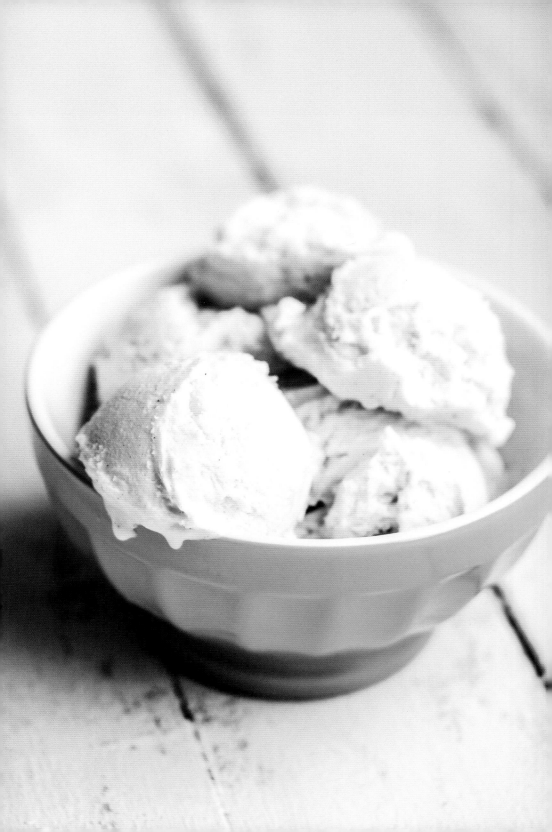

Raw Vegan Ice Cream

Prep time: 5 minutes
Cook time: 5 minutes

Ingredients
Serves 2

2 peeled frozen
bananas (freeze
overnight)

¼ cup coconut milk

Method

- Freeze peeled bananas in chunks overnight.

- Combine ingredients in food processor until thick and creamy.

- Serve immediately since it does not store well.

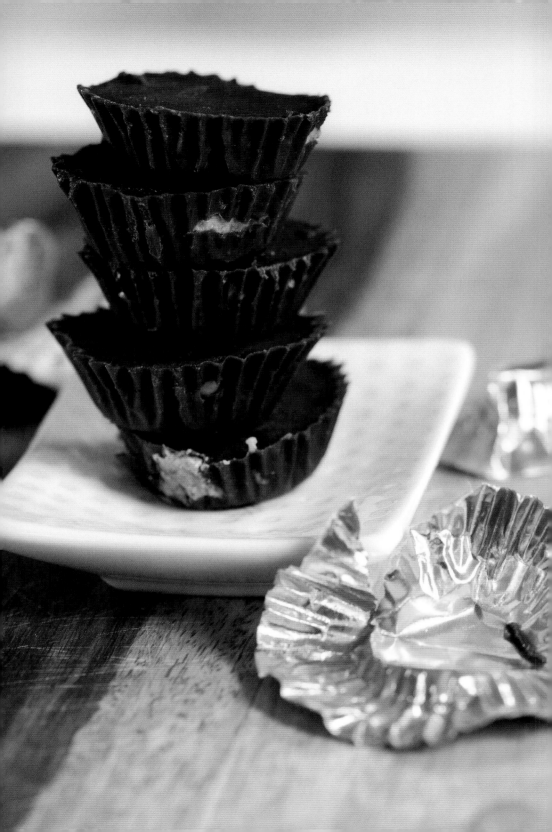

Raw Chocolate-Almond Butter Cups (V) (GF)

Prep time: 30 minutes
Cook time: 60 minutes

Ingredients
Serves 6–8

1 cup raw almonds, ground

2 tbsps raw almond butter

2 tbsps coconut oil

3 tbsps quinoa flakes, ground

2 tbsps raw honey

1 tsp vanilla extract

1 tsp fine Himalayan salt

1 cup raw cacao powder

½ cup coconut oil, melted

½ tsp vanilla extract

Method

• Whisk cacao powder into coconut oil in double boiler until smooth.

• Turn off heat and add salt and vanilla extract. Set aside in bowl.

• Grind almonds and quinoa flakes in food processor and add to bowl.

• Add coconut oil, almond butter, raw honey, vanilla extract, and salt.

• Combine well with spoon until thick paste forms.

• Line small muffin tray with paper cups.

• Drizzle one tablespoon chocolate into the bottom of each liner, then freeze for 15 minutes or until firm.

• Remove from freezer and top with one teaspoon almond mixture, then another tablespoon of chocolate.

• Return to freezer for 20–30 minutes or until mixture is firm.

• Serve immediately or store in refrigerator.

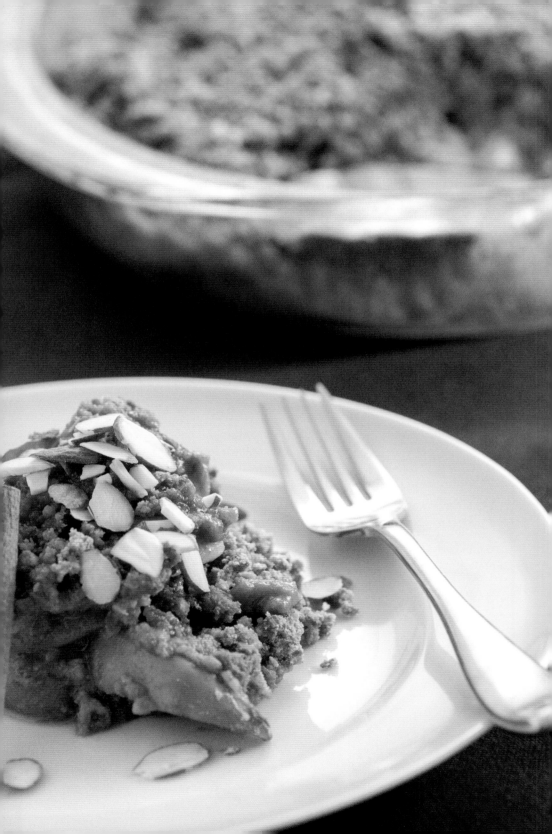

Apple-Quinoa Crumble

Prep time: 15 minutes
Cook time: 30 minutes

Ingredients
Serves 6

3 McIntosh apples

1½ cups gluten-free flour

½ cup cooked quinoa

1½ cups coconut palm sugar

¼ cup melted butter

1 egg

1 tbsp cinnamon, or to taste

Two small pinches sea salt

Method

• Preheat oven to 375°F.

• Rinse apples, peel if not organic, core, and slice into wedges.

• Toss in large bowl with ½ cup gluten-free flour, ½ cup coconut palm sugar, cinnamon, and pinch sea salt. Coat well.

• Rub a little butter in the bottom of a 10-inch diameter pie dish and arrange apples in it.

• In another large bowl, combine one cup gluten-free flour, ½ cup cooked quinoa, one cup coconut palm sugar, cinnamon, and pinch sea salt. Mix well.

• Beat egg and add to dry ingredients.

• Drizzle in melted butter and mix until crumbles form.

• Arrange crumble mixture over apples and bake for 30 minutes or until golden brown and bubbly.

Raw Fudge

Prep time: 10 minutes
Cook time: 30 minutes

Ingredients
Serves 6–8

2 cups raw cacao powder

1 cup coconut oil, melted

1 tsp vanilla extract

2 tsps fine sea salt, or to taste

Method

- Whisk cacao powder into coconut oil in double boiler until smooth.

- Turn off heat and add sea salt and vanilla extract.

- Line small muffin tray with paper cups.

- Drizzle 2 tablespoons of chocolate into each liner, then freeze for 20–30 minutes or until firm.

- Serve immediately or store in refrigerator.

Brownies

Prep time: 10 minutes
Cook time: 20 minutes

Ingredients
Serves 8–10

1 cup gluten-free flour

½ cup cocoa powder

1½ cup coconut palm sugar

2 eggs

¾ cup melted vegan butter

1 tsp pure vanilla extract

⅛ tsp sea salt, or less if your vegan butter is salted

Method

• Whisk gluten-free flour, cocoa powder, sugar, and sea salt in a large bowl.

• Melt vegan butter and add to mixture.

• Add beaten eggs and vanilla extract. Combine well.

• Rub a little bit of vegan butter in the bottom of 10 × 10 glass baking dish and pour batter in evenly.

• Bake for 20 minutes or until a knife comes out clean.

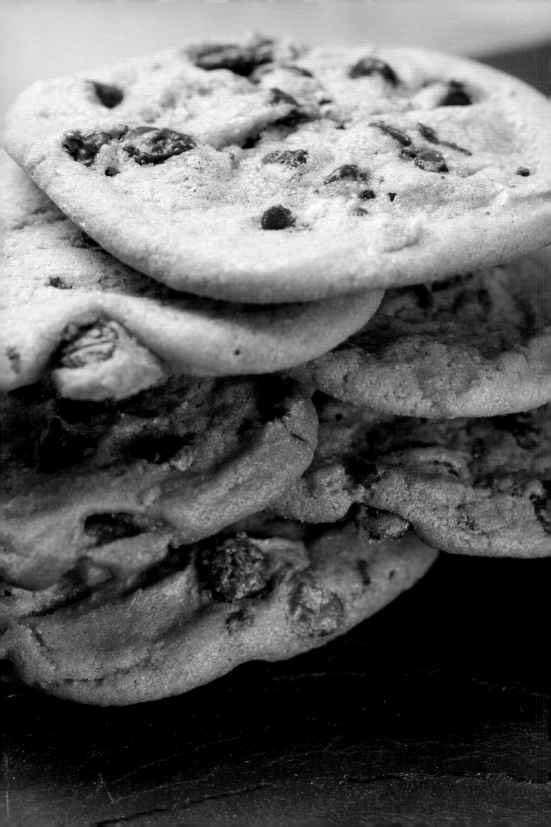

Chocolate Chip Cookies

Prep time: 10 minutes
Cook time: 15 minutes

Ingredients
Serves 10–12

1¼ cup all-purpose, whole grain, or gluten-free flour

¾ cup coconut palm sugar

½ cup butter or vegan butter at room temperature

1 egg at room temperature

½ cup dark chocolate chips

1 tsp vanilla extract

½ tsp baking soda

½ tsp baking powder

¼ tsp sea salt, or to taste

Method

• Preheat oven to 350°F.

• Combine sugar and butter or vegan butter in large bowl with electric hand mixer until creamy and fluffy.

• Beat egg in separate bowl and add, along with vanilla extract, baking soda, baking powder, and salt.

• Stir in flour and chocolate chips, combining well but not over mixing.

• Form 1-inch diameter balls and place on lined baking sheet, about 2 inches apart, and bake for 10–12 minutes, until golden brown.

• Allow to cool for 10 minutes.

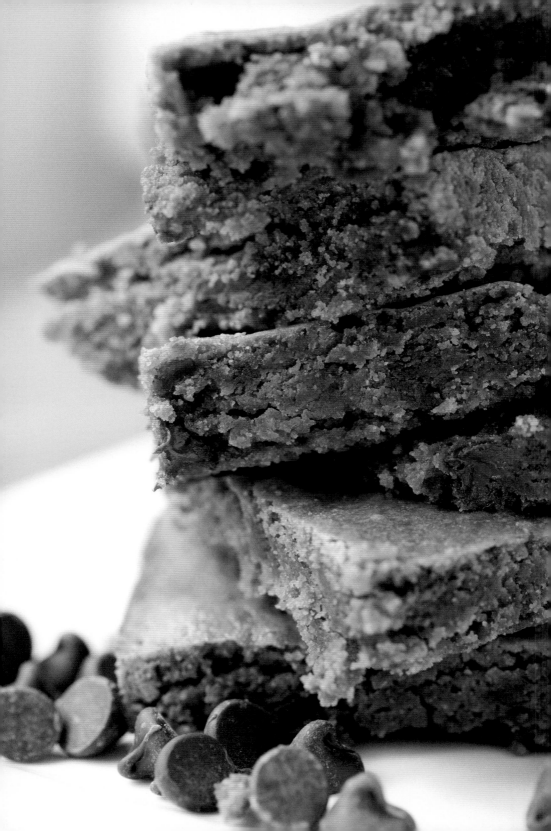

Grad Feature

Lula's Famous Dark Chocolate Blondies

Lula Brown, Class of 2013

Prep time: 10 minutes
Cook time: 30 minutes

Ingredients
Serves 8–10

1 cup gluten-free flour

1 cup coconut palm sugar

1 egg

½ cup melted vegan butter

½ cup dark chocolate chips

1 tsp pure vanilla extract

1 tsp Himalayan salt

Method

• Whisk gluten-free flour, sugar, and salt in large mixing bowl.

• Melt vegan butter and add to mixture.

• Beat egg in separate bowl and whisk in.

• Add vanilla extract and chocolate chips. Combine well.

• Rub a little bit of vegan butter in the bottom of 10 × 10 glass baking dish and pour batter in evenly.

• Bake for 30 minutes or until a knife comes out clean. Edges should be golden brown but not too dark.

·*Glossary*

I put together this glossary so you can quickly reference the benefits of different foods. Use it for yourself, your family, and/or your clients. Please note that I don't cover all the benefits of each food listed—just the most powerful ones, in my opinion. For a comprehensive list, use a search engine.

Most high-quality grocery stores stock all these items, but you may have to go to a health food store or ethnic specialty store for some. If there's not one in your area, there are great online shopping options.

You may or may not have heard of the term "primary food," which I pioneered. Primary food is the things that feed you off the plate: your career, relationships, spirituality, and exercise. When your life fulfills you, you don't need excessive food. Many people emotionally eat to try to soothe sadness or fill a deep void they feel in themselves. When you create a beautiful, exciting, full life for yourself, you don't need to overeat to feel good.

If you're an Integrative Nutrition Health Coach, please remember that it's not your job to diagnose, prescribe, or cure illnesses. Guide your clients to experiment with different foods, always under the supervision of a medical doctor.

Keep in mind that many different foods boast the same benefits, and eating a wide range of nutrient-dense foods is key to optimal health. This glossary is meant as a quick resource for you to reference specific foods, health benefits you're seeking, or conditions you're looking for nutrition support on.

Above all, focus on primary food and practical lifestyle tools with yourself, family, and clients, and you'll see much deeper transformations than if you only addressed food.

Enjoy!

Note: *This Glossary is for educational purposes and is intended to help you make informed decisions about your health. It is not intended to replace recommendations or advice from physicians or other healthcare providers. If you suspect you have a medical problem, we urge you to seek medical attention from a competent healthcare provider.*

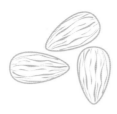

Almonds

Health Benefits	Reduce heart attack risk, lower bad cholesterol (LDL), protect artery walls, build strong bones and teeth, aid weight loss
Nutritional Information	1 oz contains 163 calories, 14g fat, 0 cholesterol, 0 sodium, 200 mg potassium, 6 g carbs, 3.5 g fiber, 1.1 g sugar
Serving Size	1 handful
Diet Specifications	

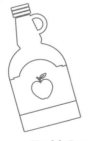

Apple Cider Vinegar

Health Benefits	Helps control diabetes and blood sugar, improves digestion and gut health, boosts immunity
Nutritional Information	1 tablespoon contains 3 calories, 0 fat, 0 cholesterol, 1 mg sodium, 11 mg potassium, 0.1 g carbs, 0 fiber, 0.1 g sugar
Serving Size	1–2 tablespoons in water
Diet Specifications	

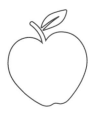

Apples

Health Benefits	Improves digestion, lowers bad cholesterol, balances blood sugar
Nutritional Information	1 medium apple contains 95 calories, 0.3 g fat, 0 cholesterol, 2 mg sodium, 195 mg potassium, 25 g carbs, 4.4 g fiber, 19 g sugar
Serving Size	1 medium apple
Diet Specifications	

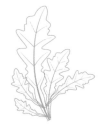

Arugula

Health Benefits	Fights inflammation, improves bone health, decreases risk of diabetes, aids digestion
Nutritional Information	½ cup contains 3 calories, 0.1 g fat, 0 cholesterol, 3 mg sodium, 37 mg potassium, 0.4 g carbs, 0.2 g fiber, 0.2 g sugar
Serving Size	½ cup
Diet Specifications	

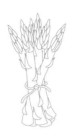

Asparagus

Health Benefits	Reduces inflammation, supports digestion, regulates blood sugar, improves heart health
Nutritional Information	1 cup contains 27 calories, 0.2 g fat, 0 cholesterol, 3 mg sodium, 271 mg potassium, 5 g carbs, 2.8 g fiber, 2.5 g sugar
Serving Size	1 cup
Diet Specifications	

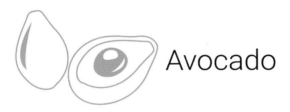

Avocado

Health Benefits	Supports heart health, lowers cholesterol levels, improves digestive and skin health
Nutritional Information	1 avocado contains 322 calories, 29 g fat, 0 cholesterol, 14 mg sodium, 975 mg potassium, 17 g carbs, 14 g fiber, 1.3 g sugar, 4 g protein
Serving Size	¼ avocado
Diet Specifications	

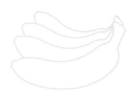

Bananas

Health Benefits	Supports digestion and circulation, lowers blood pressure, reduces inflammation, improves heart health
Nutritional Information	1 medium banana contains 105 calories, 0.4 g fat, 0 mg cholesterol, 1 mg sodium, 422 mg potassium, 27 g carbs, 3.1 g fiber, 14 g sugar, 1.3 g protein
Serving Size	1 medium banana
Diet Specifications	GF VG V

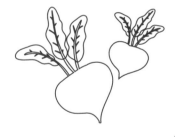

Beets

Health Benefits	Improves blood quality and flow, cleanses the body, improves mental function, boosts libido
Nutritional Information	1 cup contains 59 calories, 0.2 g fat, 0 cholesterol, 106 mg sodium, 442 mg potassium, 13 g carbs, 3.8 g fiber, 9 g sugar, 2.2 g protein
Serving Size	1 cup
Diet Specifications	GF VG V

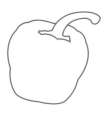

Bell Peppers

Health Benefits	Improves immunity, reduces inflammation, supports skin and hair health, protects eye health
Nutritional Information	1 medium bell pepper contains 24 calories, 0.2 g fat, 0 cholesterol, 4 mg sodium, 208 mg potassium, 6 g carbs, 2 g fiber, 2.9 g sugar, 1 g protein
Serving Size	1 medium bell pepper
Diet Specifications	

Blackberries

Health Benefits	Reduces inflammation, improves mental function, aids digestion, boosts heart health, aids weight loss
Nutritional Information	1 cup contains 62 calories, 0.7 g fat, 0 cholesterol, 1 mg sodium, 233 mg potassium, 14 g carbs, 8 g fiber, 7 g sugar, 2 g protein
Serving Size	1 cup
Diet Specifications	

Blueberries

Health Benefits	Aids digestion, boosts immunity, fights inflammation, decreases the risk of heart disease
Nutritional Information	1 cup contains 85 calories, 0.5 g fat, 0 cholesterol, 1 mg sodium, 114 mg potassium, 21 g carbs, 3.6 g fiber, 15 g sugar, 1.1 g protein
Serving Size	1 cup
Diet Specifications	

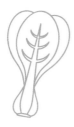

Bok Choy

Health Benefits	Aids digestion, reduces blood pressure, increases metabolism, reduces inflammation
Nutritional Information	1 cup shredded contains 9 calories, 0.1 g fat, 0 cholesterol, 46 mg sodium, 176 mg potassium, 1.5 g carbs, 0.7 g fiber, 0.8 g sugar, 1 g protein
Serving Size	1 cup shredded
Diet Specifications	

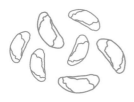

Brazil Nuts

Health Benefits	Improves focus, promotes satiety, boosts immunity and thyroid function, decrea ses the risk of heart disease; an excellent source of selenium, which contributes to healthy thyroid metabolism and protects the body from oxidative damage and stress
Nutritional Information	1 oz contains 186 calories, 19 g fat, 0 cholesterol, 1 mg sodium, 187 mg potassium, 3.5 g carbs, 2.1 g fiber, 0.7 g sugar, 4.1 g protein
Serving Size	6 nuts
Diet Specifications	

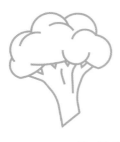

Broccoli

Health Benefits	Aids digestion, reduces inflammation, detoxifies the body, supports heart health
Nutritional Information	1 cup chopped contains 31 calories, 0.3 g fat, 0 cholesterol, 30 mg sodium, 288 mg potassium, 6 g carbs, 2.4 g fiber, 1.6 g sugar, 2.6 g protein
Serving Size	1 cup chopped
Diet Specifications	

Brussels Sprouts

Health Benefits	Improves immunity, aids digestion, supports weight loss, improves focus, fights inflammation
Nutritional Information	1 cup contains 38 calories, 0 fat, 0 cholesterol, 22 mg sodium, 342 mg potassium, 8 g carbs, 3 g fiber, 2 g sugar, 3 g protein
Serving Size	1 cup
Diet Specifications	V

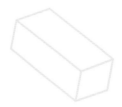

Butter

Health Benefits	Improves focus, supports skin health, reduces risk of heart disease, improves good cholesterol; grass-fed varieties of butter contain higher levels of omega 3's and 6's
Nutritional Information	1 tablespoon contains 102 calories, 12 g fat, 31 mg cholesterol, 2 mg sodium, 3 mg potassium, 0 g carbs, 0 g fiber, 0 g sugar, 0.1 g protein
Serving Size	1 tablespoon
Diet Specifications	

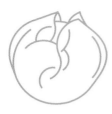

Cabbage

Health Benefits	Lowers bad cholesterol, stabilizes blood sugar, prevents inflammation, aids digestion
Nutritional Information	1 cup chopped contains 22 calories, 0 fat, 0 cholesterol, 16 mg sodium, 151 mg potassium, 5 g carbs, 2 g fiber, 3 g sugar, 1 g protein
Serving Size	1 cup chopped
Diet Specifications	

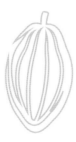

Cacao

Health Benefits	Improves digestion and circulation, reduces inflammation, improves blood and bone health
Nutritional Information	1 tablespoon raw powder contains 20 calories, 0.5 g fat, 0 cholesterol, 0 sodium, 87 mg potassium, 3 g carbs, 1 g fiber, 0 sugar, 1 g protein
Serving Size	1 tablespoon
Diet Specifications	

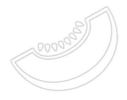

Cantaloupe

Health Benefits	Reduces inflammation, aids digestion, improves vision, lowers risk of metabolic syndrome
Nutritional Information	1 cup diced contains 53 calories, 0.3 g fat, 0 cholesterol, 25 mg sodium, 417 mg potassium, 13 g carbs, 1.4 g fiber, 12 g sugar, 1.3 g protein
Serving Size	1 cup diced
Diet Specifications	V

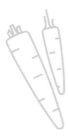

Carrots

Health Benefits	Improves eye health, aids digestion, balances blood sugar, improves immunity
Nutritional Information	1 medium carrot contains 25 calories, 0 fat, 0 cholesterol, 42 mg sodium, 195 mg potassium, 6 g carbs, 1.7 g fiber, 2.9 g sugar, 1 g protein
Serving Size	1 medium carrot
Diet Specifications	

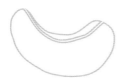

Cashews

Health Benefits	Protects heart health, increases energy, boosts brain function, supports bone and blood health
Nutritional Information	1 oz contains 157 calories, 12 g fat, 0 cholesterol, 3 mg sodium, 187 mg potassium, 9 g carbs, 1 g fiber, 2 g sugar, 5 g protein
Serving Size	16 nuts
Diet Specifications	

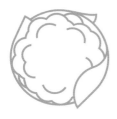

Cauliflower

Health Benefits	Boosts immunity, aids digestion, reduces inflammation, balances blood sugar
Nutritional Information	1 cup contains 25 calories, 0 fat, 0 cholesterol, 30 mg sodium, 303 mg potassium, 5 g carbs, 3 g fiber, 2 g sugar, 2 g protein
Serving Size	1 cup
Diet Specifications	

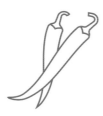

Cayenne

Health Benefits	Improves immunity, decreases candida, improves circulation, supports detoxification, aids weight loss
Nutritional Information	1 teaspoon contains 6 calories, 0 fat, 0 cholesterol, 1 mg sodium, 36 mg potassium, 1 g carbs, 1 g fiber, 0 sugar, 0 protein
Serving Size	1 teaspoon
Diet Specifications	

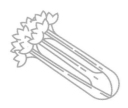

Celery

Health Benefits	Supports healthy vision, boosts immunity, alkalizes the body, builds bone health, aids digestion
Nutritional Information	2 stalks contain 18 calories, 0 fat, 0 cholesterol, 88 mg sodium, 286 mg potassium, 3 g carbs, 2 g fiber, 2 g sugar, 1 g protein
Serving Size	2 stalks
Diet Specifications	

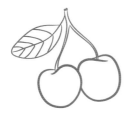

Cherries

Health Benefits	Prevents inflammation, reduces supports weight loss, improves sleep quality, reduces muscle pain
Nutritional Information	1 cup contains 77 calories, 1 g fat, 0 cholesterol, 5 mg sodium, 268 mg potassium, 19 g carbs, 3 g fiber, 13 g sugar, 2 g protein
Serving Size	1 cup
Diet Specifications	V

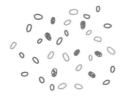

Chia Seeds

Health Benefits	Aids digestion, supports high energy, accelerates weight loss, improves brain function, balances blood sugar
Nutritional Information	2 tablespoons contain 138 calories, 9 g fat, 0 cholesterol, 5 mg sodium, 115 mg potassium, 12 g carbs, 10 g fiber, 0 sugar, 5 g protein
Serving Size	2 tablespoons
Diet Specifications	

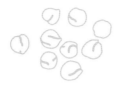

Chickpeas

Health Benefits	Regulates appetite, supports weight loss, aids digestion, balances blood sugar, reduces cholesterol
Nutritional Information	1 cup contains 269 calories, 4 g fat, 0 cholesterol, 11 mg sodium, 477 mg potassium, 45 g carbs, 12 g fiber, 8 g sugar, 15 g protein
Serving Size	1 cup
Diet Specifications	V

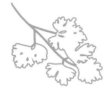

Cilantro

Health Benefits	Promotes detoxification, fights candida, boosts immunity, reduces inflammation, supports bone health
Nutritional Information	¼ cup contains 1 calorie, 0 fat, 0 cholesterol, 2 mg sodium, 21 mg potassium, 0 carbs, 0 fiber, 0 sugar, 0 protein
Serving Size	¼ cup
Diet Specifications	

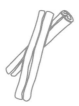

Cinnamon

Health Benefits	Improves circulation, aids digestion, balances appetite, protects against heart disease
Nutritional Information	1 teaspoon contains 6 calories, 0 fat, 0 cholesterol, 0 sodium, 11 mg potassium, 2 g carbs, 1 g fiber, 0 sugar, 0 protein
Serving Size	1 teaspoon
Diet Specifications	

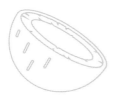

Coconut Meat

Health Benefits	Supports weight loss, improves mental function, fights candida, improves immunity
Nutritional Information	1 cup shredded contains 283 calories, 27 g fat, 0 cholesterol, 16 mg sodium, 285 mg potassium, 12 g carbs, 7 g fiber, 5 g sugar, 3 g protein
Serving Size	1 cup shredded
Diet Specifications	

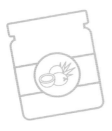

Coconut Oil

Health Benefits	Supports weight loss, improves mental function, fights candida, improves immunity
Nutritional Information	1 tablespoon contains 117 calories, 14 g fat, 0 cholesterol, 0 sodium, 0 potassium, 0 carbs, 0 fiber, 0 sugar, 0 protein
Serving Size	1 tablespoon
Diet Specifications	

Coconut Palm Sugar

Health Benefits	Balances blood sugar, increases energy
Nutritional Information	1 teaspoon contains 15 calories, 0 fat, 0 cholesterol, 5 mg sodium, 24 mg potassium, 4 g carbs, 0 fiber, 4 g sugar, 0 protein
Serving Size	1 teaspoon
Diet Specifications	

Coffee

Health Benefits	Increases energy, helps prevents diabetes, lowers the risk of liver disease, reduces inflammation
Nutritional Information	1 cup contains 1 calorie, 0 fat, 0 cholesterol, 5 mg sodium, 116 mg potassium, 0 carbs, 0 fiber, 0 sugar, 0 protein
Serving Size	8 ounces
Diet Specifications	

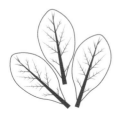

Collard Greens

Health Benefits	Improves digestion, increases energy, detoxifies the body, stabilizes blood sugar
Nutritional Information	1 cup contains 11 calories, 0 fat, 0 cholesterol, 6 mg sodium, 77 mg potassium, 2 g carbs, 1.4 g fiber, 0 sugar, 1 g protein
Serving Size	1 cup
Diet Specifications	

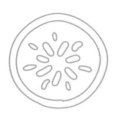

Cucumbers

Health Benefits	Hydrates and cools the body, boosts skin health, aids weight loss, supports eye health
Nutritional Information	½ cup contains 8 calories, 0 fat, 0 cholesterol, 1 mg sodium, 76 mg potassium, 2 g carbs, 0 fiber, 1 g sugar, 0 protein
Serving Size	½ cup sliced
Diet Specifications	V

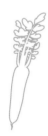

Daikon Radish

Health Benefits	Burns fat, boosts immunity, fights inflammation, aids digestion, detoxifies the body
Nutritional Information	1 radish contains 61 calories, 0 fat, 0 cholesterol, 71 mg sodium, 767 mg potassium, 14 g carbs, 5 g fiber, 8 g sugar, 2 g protein
Serving Size	1 radish
Diet Specifications	V

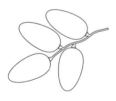

Dates

Health Benefits	Improves digestion, reduces the risk of anemia, improves sexual function, increases circulation
Nutritional Information	½ cup dates contains 251 calories, 0 fat, 0 cholesterol, 2 mg sodium, 584 mg potassium, 67 g carbs, 7 g fiber, 56 g sugar, 2 g protein
Serving Size	½ cup
Diet Specifications	GF VG V

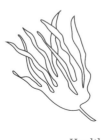

Dulse

Health Benefits	Alkalizes the body, aids detoxification, supports brain function, improves thyroid health
Nutritional Information	1 tablespoon contains 13 calories, 0 fat, 0 cholesterol, 85 mg sodium, 383 mg potassium, 2 g carbs, 2 g fiber, 0 sugar, 1 g protein
Serving Size	1 tablespoon
Diet Specifications	GF VG V

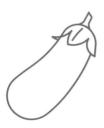

Eggplant

Health Benefits	Aids digestion, supports adrenal health, reduces anxiety, fights inflammation, supports brain health
Nutritional Information	1 cup contains 20 calories, 0 fat, 0 cholesterol, 2 mg sodium, 188 mg potassium, 5 g carbs, 3 g fiber, 3 g sugar, 1 g protein
Serving Size	1 cup cubes
Diet Specifications	

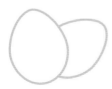

Eggs

Health Benefits	Improves brain function, balances blood sugar, supports weight loss, supports adrenal health
Nutritional Information	2 eggs contain 147 calories, 10 g fat, 423 mg cholesterol, 140 mg sodium, 134 mg potassium, 1 g carbs, 0 fiber, 1 g sugar, 13 g protein
Serving Size	2 eggs
Diet Specifications	

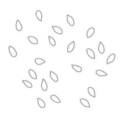

Flaxseeds

Health Benefits	Promotes heart health, improves brain function, balances hormones, reduces inflammation
Nutritional Information	1 clove contains 4 calories, 0 fat, 0 cholesterol, 1 mg sodium, 12 mg potassium, 1 g carbs, 0 fiber, 0 sugar, 0 protein
Serving Size	1 clove
Diet Specifications	

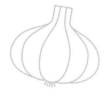

Garlic

Health Benefits	Improves immunity, reduces blood pressure, lowers the risk of heart disease, supports detoxification
Nutritional Information	1 clove contains 4 calories, 0 fat, 0 cholesterol, 1 mg sodium, 12 mg potassium, 1 g carbs, 0 fiber, 0 sugar, 0 protein
Serving Size	1 clove
Diet Specifications	

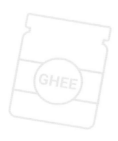

Ghee

Health Benefits	Improves brain function, supports digestion, boosts skin health, maintains healthy vision
Nutritional Information	1 tablespoon contains 112 calories, 13 g fat, 33 mg cholesterol, 0 sodium, 1 mg potassium, 0 carbs, 0 fiber, 0 sugar, 0 protein
Serving Size	1 tablespoon
Diet Specifications	

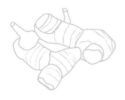

Ginger

Health Benefits	Treats nausea and motion sickness, improves digestion, boosts immunity, promotes cell growth
Nutritional Information	1 teaspoon contains 2 calories, 0 fat, 0 cholesterol, 0 sodium, 11 mg potassium, 0 carbs, 0 fiber, 0 sugar, 0 protein
Serving Size	1 teaspoon grated
Diet Specifications	

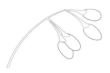

Goji Berries

Health Benefits	Reduces diabetes and hypertension, improves immunity, protects eye health, improves digestion
Nutritional Information	2 tablespoons contain 23 calories, 0 fat, 0 cholesterol, 7 mg sodium, 0 potassium, 6 g carbs, 2 g fiber, 4 g sugar, 3 g protein
Serving Size	2 tablespoons
Diet Specifications	

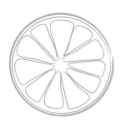

Grapefruit

Health Benefits	Boosts immunity, improves digestion, aids nausea, lowers cholesterol, reduces risk of kidney stones
Nutritional Information	½ grapefruit contains 52 calories, 0 fat, 0 cholesterol, 0 sodium, 166 mg potassium, 13 g carbs, 2 g fiber, 8 g sugar, 1 g protein
Serving Size	½ grapefruit
Diet Specifications	

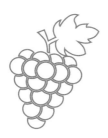

Grapes

Health Benefits	Improves immunity, supports cardiovascular health, balances blood sugar, improves brain health
Nutritional Information	1 cup contains 104 calories, 0 fat, 0 cholesterol, 3 mg sodium, 176 mg potassium, 27 g carbs, 1 g fiber, 23 g sugar, 1 g protein
Serving Size	1 cup
Diet Specifications	

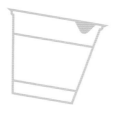

Greek Yogurt

Health Benefits	Regulates blood sugar, improves muscle mass, supports digestive regularity, improves bone health
Nutritional Information	1 cup contains 190 calories, 10 g fat, 25 mg cholesterol, 70 mg sodium, 420 mg potassium, 8 g carbs, 0 fiber, 8 g sugar, 18 g protein
Serving Size	1 cup
Diet Specifications	

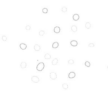

Hemp Seeds

Health Benefits	Supports brain health, aids weight loss, improves digestion, balances blood sugar, improves cholesterol levels
Nutritional Information	3 tablespoons contain 170 calories, 14 g fat, 0 cholesterol, 0 sodium, 360 mg potassium, 2 g carbs, 1 g fiber, 0 g sugar, 10 g protein
Serving Size	3 tablespoons
Diet Specifications	

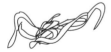

Hijiki

Health Benefits	Improves hair, skin, and nail health, boosts mental function, balances hormones
Nutritional Information	1 teaspoon contains 0 calories, 0 fat, 0 cholesterol, 15 mg sodium, 50 mg potassium, 0 carbs, 1 g fiber, 0 sugar, 0 protein
Serving Size	1 teaspoon
Diet Specifications	

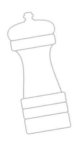

Himalayan Salt

Health Benefits	Balances blood sugar, reduces signs of aging, improves hydration, supports libido
Nutritional Information	1 teaspoon contains 0 calories, 0 fat, 0 cholesterol, 2325 mg sodium, 0 potassium, 0 carbs, 0 fiber, 0 sugar, 0 protein
Serving Size	¼ teaspoon
Diet Specifications	

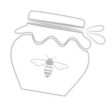

Honey

Health Benefits	Reduces allergic reactions, improves memory, heals wounds and burns, improves sleep quality
Nutritional Information	1 tablespoon contains 64 calories, 0 fat, 0 cholesterol, 1 mg sodium, 11 mg potassium, 17 g carbs, 0 fiber, 17 g sugar, 0 protein
Serving Size	1 tablespoon
Diet Specifications	

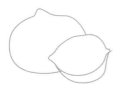

Jicama

Health Benefits	Improves digestion, stabilizes blood sugar, improves immunity, supports adrenal health, reduces anxiety
Nutritional Information	1 cup of jicama contains 49 calories, 0 fat, 0 cholesterol, 5 mg sodium, 195 mg potassium, 11 g carbs, 6 g fiber, 2 g sugar, 1 g protein
Serving Size	1 cup
Diet Specifications	

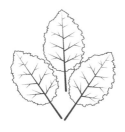

Kale

Health Benefits	Improves digestion, fights inflammation, improves immunity, lowers cholesterol, protects against heart disease
Nutritional Information	1 cup contains 33 calories, 1 g fat, 0 cholesterol, 25 mg sodium, 329 mg potassium, 6 g carbs, 3 g fiber, 2 g sugar, 3 g protein
Serving Size	1 cup
Diet Specifications	

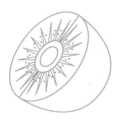

Kiwi

Health Benefits	Improves immunity, facilitates digestion, balances blood sugar, protects heart and eye health
Nutritional Information	1 fruit contains 42 calories, 0 fat, 0 cholesterol, 2 mg sodium, 215 mg potassium, 10 g carbs, 2 g fiber, 6 g sugar, 1 g protein
Serving Size	1 fruit
Diet Specifications	GF VG V

Lemons

Health Benefits	Aids digestion, supports weight loss, reduces blood pressure, detoxes the body, improves immunity
Nutritional Information	1 fruit contains 17 calories, 0 fat, 0 cholesterol, 1 mg sodium, 80 mg potassium, 5 g carbs, 2 g fiber, 1 g sugar, 1 g protein
Serving Size	Juice of 1 fruit
Diet Specifications	GF VG V

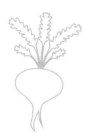

Maca

Health Benefits	Increases libido, improves digestion, reduces PMS, balances mood, increases energy, improves skin health
Nutritional Information	2 tablespoons contain 50 calories, 0 fat, 0 cholesterol, 3 mg sodium, 219 mg potassium, 10 g carbs, 3 g fiber, 4 g sugar, 2 g protein
Serving Size	2 tablespoons
Diet Specifications	

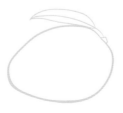

Mango

Health Benefits	Protects against inflammation, improves digestion, balances blood sugar, improves skin health, boosts immunity
Nutritional Information	1 mango contains 201 calories, 1 g fat, 0 cholesterol, 3 mg sodium, 564 mg potassium, 50 g carbs, 5 g fiber, 46 g sugar, 3 g protein
Serving Size	1 mango
Diet Specifications	

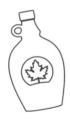

Maple Syrup

Health Benefits	Reduces inflammation, boosts immune system, improves digestion and soothes nausea, reduces bloating
Nutritional Information	1 tablespoon contains 52 calories, 0 fat, 0 cholesterol, 2 mg sodium, 42 mg potassium, 13 g carbs, 0 fiber, 14 g sugar, 0 protein
Serving Size	1 tablespoon
Diet Specifications	V

Mint

Health Benefits	Eases indigestion, fights inflammation, antimicrobial, improves immunity, improves mental focus
Nutritional Information	2 tablespoons contain 2 calories, 0 fat, 0 cholesterol, 1 mg sodium, 18 mg potassium, 0 carbs, 0 fiber, 0 sugar, 0 protein
Serving Size	2 tablespoons chopped
Diet Specifications	

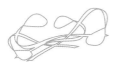

Mung Bean Sprouts

Health Benefits	Improves blood health, supports bone health, improves immunity, supports skin health, improves circulation
Nutritional Information	1 cup contains 31 calories, 0 fat, 0 cholesterol, 6 mg sodium, 155 mg potassium, 6 g carbs, 2 g fiber, 4 g sugar, 3 g protein
Serving Size	1 cup
Diet Specifications	

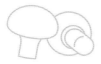

Mushrooms

Health Benefits	Supports weight loss, improves immunity, prevents strokes, regulates blood pressure, protects heart health
Nutritional Information	1 cup contains 21 calories, 0 fat, 0 cholesterol, 5 mg sodium, 273 mg potassium, 4 g carbs, 2 g fiber, 1 g sugar, 1 g protein
Serving Size	1 cup
Diet Specifications	

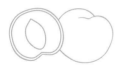

Nectarines

Health Benefits	Improves digestion, stabilizes blood sugar, supports cardiovascular health, aids weight loss, improves skin health
Nutritional Information	1 medium fruit contains 59 calories, 0 fat, 0 cholesterol, 0 sodium, 285 mg potassium, 14 g carbs, 2 g fiber, 13 g sugar, 1 g protein
Serving Size	1 medium fruit
Diet Specifications	

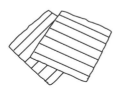

Nori

Health Benefits	Stabilizes blood sugar, lowers cholesterol, improves digestion, boosts mental focus, supports thyroid health, balances hormones
Nutritional Information	2 tablespoons contain 4 calories, 0 fat, 0 cholesterol, 5 mg sodium, 36 mg potassium, 1 g carbs, 0 fiber, 0 sugar, 1 g protein
Serving Size	2 tablespoons shredded
Diet Specifications	

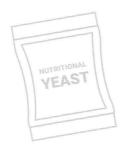

Nutritional Yeast

Health Benefits	Supports adrenal health, reduces stress, supports weight loss, builds and repairs muscles
Nutritional Information	2 tablespoons contain 79 calories, 1 g fat, 0 cholesterol, 9 mg sodium, 320 mg potassium, 9 g carbs, 7 g fiber, 2 g sugar, 14 g protein
Serving Size	2 tablespoons
Diet Specifications	

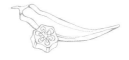

Okra

Health Benefits	Facilitates digestion, balances blood sugar, reduces the risk of heart disease, supports weight loss
Nutritional Information	1 cup contains 33 calories, 0 fat, 0 cholesterol, 7 mg sodium, 299 mg potassium, 7 g carbs, 3 g fiber, 2 g sugar, 2 g protein
Serving Size	1 cup
Diet Specifications	

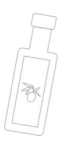

Olive Oil

Health Benefits	Lowers cholesterol, protects heart health, improves mental focus, supports weight loss, supports bone health
Nutritional Information	1 tablespoon contains 119 calories, 14 g fat, 0 cholesterol, 0 sodium, 0 potassium, 0 carbs, 0 fiber, 0 sugar, 0 protein
Serving Size	1 tablespoon
Diet Specifications	

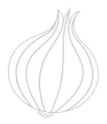

Onions

Health Benefits	Balances blood sugar, improves immunity, protects heart health, supports bone and tissue health
Nutritional Information	1 medium onion contains 44 calories, 0 fat, 0 cholesterol, 4 mg sodium, 161 mg potassium, 10 g carbs, 2 g fiber, 5 g sugar, 1 g protein
Serving Size	1 medium onion
Diet Specifications	

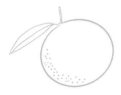

Oranges

Health Benefits	Improves immunity, supports heart health, improves digestion, protects respiratory health
Nutritional Information	1 fruit contains 62 calories, 0 fat, 0 cholesterol, 0 sodium, 237 mg potassium, 15 g carbs, 3 g fiber, 12 g sugar, 1 g protein
Serving Size	1 fruit
Diet Specifications	

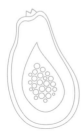

Papayas

Health Benefits	Improves digestion, supports skin health, boosts immunity, protects vision, supports healthy muscles
Nutritional Information	1 small fruit contains 67 calories, 0 fat, 0 cholesterol, 13 mg sodium, 286 mg potassium, 17 g carbs, 3 g fiber, 12 g sugar, 1 g proteins
Serving Size	1 small fruit
Diet Specifications	

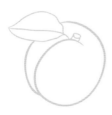

Peaches

Health Benefits	Supports weight loss, balances blood sugar, improves digestion, balances blood pressure
Nutritional Information	1 medium fruit contains 59 calories, 0 fat, 0 cholesterol, 0 sodium, 285 mg potassium, 14 g carbs, 2 g fiber, 13 g sugar, 1 g protein
Serving Size	1 medium fruit
Diet Specifications	GF VG V

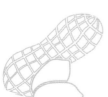

Peanuts

Health Benefits	Protect heart health, balances blood sugar, improves boosts energy and mental focus
Nutritional Information	1 ounce contains 161 calories, 14 g fat, 0 cholesterol, 5 mg sodium, 200 mg potassium, 5 g carbs, 2 g fiber, 1 g sugar, 7 g protein
Serving Size	1 handful
Diet Specifications	GF VG V

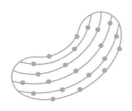

Pickles

Health Benefits	Improves gut health, reduces anxiety, improves immunity, protects against infection, curbs appetite
Nutritional Information	1 pickle contains 8 calories, 0 fat, 0 cholesterol, 569 mg sodium, 60 mg potassium, 2 g carbs, 1 g fiber, 1 g sugar, 0 protein
Serving Size	1 pickle
Diet Specifications	

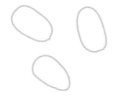

Pine Nuts

Health Benefits	Balances cholesterol levels, boosts energy, regulates appetite, balances blood sugar, supports healthy aging
Nutritional Information	1 ounce contains 191 calories, 19 g fat, 0 cholesterol, 1 mg sodium, 169 mg potassium, 4 g carbs, 1 g fiber, 1 g sugar, 4 g protein
Serving Size	1 palmful
Diet Specifications	

Pineapple

Health Benefits	Burns fat, improves immunity, aids digestion, eases muscle soreness, supports eye health
Nutritional Information	1 cup contains 82 calories, 0 fat, 0 cholesterol, 2 mg sodium, 180 mg potassium, 22 g carbs, 2 g fiber, 16 g sugar, 1 g protein
Serving Size	1 cup cubes
Diet Specifications	

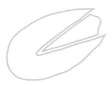

Pistachios

Health Benefits	Stabilizes blood sugar, supports weight loss, boosts brain health, improves healthy cholesterol levels
Nutritional Information	1 ounce contains 159 calories, 13 g fat, 0 cholesterol, 0 sodium, 291 mg potassium, 8 g carbs, 3 g fiber, 2 g sugar, 6 g protein
Serving Size	1 palmful
Diet Specifications	

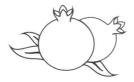

Pomegranates

Health Benefits	Fights inflammation, protects heart health, boosts immunity, lowers blood pressure, fights osteoporosis
Nutritional Information	½ cup seeds contains 72 calories, 1 g fat, 0 cholesterol, 3 mg sodium, 205 mg potassium, 16 g carbs, 3.5 g fiber, 12 g sugar, 1 g protein
Serving Size	½ cup seeds
Diet Specifications	

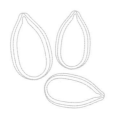

Pumpkin Seeds

Health Benefits	Fights inflammation, improves focus, balances blood sugar, supports weight loss, improves immunity
Nutritional Information	1 ounce contains 126 calories, 6 g fat, 0 cholesterol, 5 mg sodium, 261 mg potassium, 15 g carbs, 5 g fiber, 0 sugar, 5 g protein
Serving Size	1 palmful
Diet Specifications	

Raspberries

Health Benefits	Boosts immunity, improves digestion, protects heart health, supports healthy aging, reduces inflammation
Nutritional Information	1 cup contains 65 calories, 1 g fat, 0 cholesterol, 1 mg sodium, 186 mg potassium, 15 g carbs, 8 g fiber, 5 g sugar, 2 g protein
Serving Size	1 cup
Diet Specifications	V

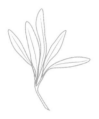

Sage

Health Benefits	Improves digestion, supports cognitive function, wards off chronic disease, improves memory, balances blood sugar
Nutritional Information	1 teaspoon contains 2 calories, 0 fat, 0 cholesterol, 0 sodium, 7 mg potassium, 0 carbs, 0 fiber, 0 sugar, 0 protein
Serving Size	1 teaspoon chopped
Diet Specifications	

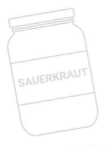

Sauerkraut

Health Benefits	Improves digestion, supports weight loss, improves cognitive function, increases immunity, improves absorption
Nutritional Information	100 grams contains 19 calories, 0 fat, 0 cholesterol, 661 mg sodium, 170 mg potassium, 4 g carbs, 3 g fiber, 2 g sugar, 1 g protein
Serving Size	3 tablespoons
Diet Specifications	

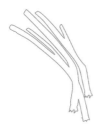

Scallions

Health Benefits	Improves digestion, supports weight loss, improves immunity, supports adrenal health
Nutritional Information	1 medium scallion contains 5 calories, 0 fat, 0 cholesterol, 2 mg sodium, 41 mg potassium, 1 g carbs, 0 fiber, 0 sugar, 0 protein
Serving Size	1 tablespoon chopped
Diet Specifications	

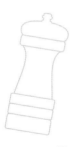

Sea Salt

Health Benefits	Regulates blood pressure, improves hydration, increases absorption, supports digestion, improves bone health
Nutritional Information	¼ teaspoon contains 0 calories, 0 fat, 0 cholesterol, 590 mg sodium, 0 potassium, 0 carbs, 0 fiber, 0 sugar, 0 protein
Serving Size	¼ teaspoon
Diet Specifications	

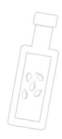

Sesame Oil

Health Benefits	Lowers blood pressure, improves focus, supports weight loss, balances blood sugar, improves skin health
Nutritional Information	1 tablespoon contains 120 calories, 14 g fat, 0 cholesterol, 0 sodium, 0 potassium, 0 carbs, 0 fiber, 0 sugar, 0 protein
Serving Size	1 tablespoon
Diet Specifications	

Sesame Seeds

Health Benefits	Improves energy levels, supports liver, heart, kidney, and brain health, improves skeletal muscle health
Nutritional Information	1 tablespoon contains 52 calories, 5 g fat, 0 cholesterol, 1 mg sodium, 42 mg potassium, 2 g carbs, 1 g fiber, 0 sugar, 2 g protein
Serving Size	1 tablespoon
Diet Specifications	

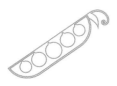

Snap Peas

Health Benefits	Improves digestion, balances blood sugar, reduces sugar cravings, improves bone health, boosts energy
Nutritional Information	1 cup contain 41 calories, 0 fat, 0 cholesterol, 4 mg sodium, 196 mg potassium, 7 g carbs, 3 g fiber, 4 g sugar, 3 g protein
Serving Size	1 cup
Diet Specifications	

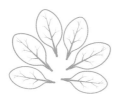

Spinach

Health Benefits	Improves bone, skin, and hair health, supports digestion, maintains bone health
Nutritional Information	1 cup contains 7 calories, 0 fat, 0 cholesterol, 24 mg sodium, 167 mg potassium, 1 g carbs, 1 g fiber, 0 sugar, 1 g protein
Serving Size	1 cup
Diet Specifications	

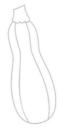

Squash (Butternut)

Health Benefits	Improves digestion, balances blood sugar, reduces inflammation, supports heart health
Nutritional Information	1 cup contains 63 calories, 0 fat, 0 cholesterol, 6 mg sodium, 493 mg potassium, 16 g carbs, 3 g fiber, 3 g sugar, 1 g protein
Serving Size	1 cup cubes
Diet Specifications	

Stevia

Health Benefits	Supports weight loss, lowers risk of obesity and diabetes, reduces sugar consumption, maintains mood
Nutritional Information	½ teaspoon contains 0 calories, 0 fat, 0 cholesterol, 0 sodium, 0 potassium, 0 carbs, 0 fiber, 0 sugar, 0 protein
Serving Size	½ teaspoon
Diet Specifications	V

Strawberries

Health Benefits	Improves immunity, supports cardiovascular health, reduces inflammation, balances blood sugar
Nutritional Information	1 cup contains 54 calories, 1 g fat, 0 cholesterol, 2 mg sodium, 254 mg potassium, 13 g carbs, 3 g fiber, 8 g sugar, 1 g protein
Serving Size	1 cup
Diet Specifications	

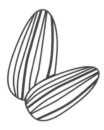

Sunflower Seeds

Health Benefits	Lowers risk of cardiovascular disease and type 2 diabetes, improves skin health, lowers cholesterol
Nutritional Information	1 ounce contains 165 calories, 14 g fat, 0 cholesterol, 1 mg sodium, 241 mg potassium, 7 g carbs, 3 g fiber, 1 g sugar, 5 g protein
Serving Size	1 palmful
Diet Specifications	

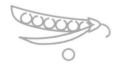

Sweet Peas

Health Benefits	Reduces inflammation, regulates blood sugar, promotes heart health, improves digestion
Nutritional Information	1 cup contains 118 calories, 1 g fat, 0 cholesterol, 7 mg sodium, 354 mg potassium, 21 g carbs, 7 g fiber, 8 g sugar, 8 g protein
Serving Size	1 cup
Diet Specifications	V

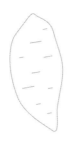

Sweet Potato

Health Benefits	Improves digestion, stabilizes blood sugar, improves skin health, reduces inflammation
Nutritional Information	1 medium sweet potato contains 112 calories, 0 fat, 0 cholesterol, 72 mg sodium, 438 mg potassium, 26 g carbs, 4 g fiber, 5 g sugar, 2 g protein
Serving Size	1 medium sweet potato
Diet Specifications	V

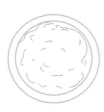

Tahini

Health Benefits	Supports brain health, aids weight loss, balances blood sugar, maintains skin and muscle health
Nutritional Information	1 tablespoon contains 89 calories, 8 g fat, 0 cholesterol, 17 mg sodium, 62 mg potassium, 3 g carbs, 1 g fiber, 0 sugar, 3 g protein
Serving Size	1 tablespoon
Diet Specifications	

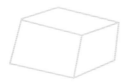

Tofu

Health Benefits	Protects heart health, lowers risk of type 2 diabetes, stabilizes blood sugar, supports bone health
Nutritional Information	½ cup contains 94 calories, 6 g fat, 0 cholesterol, 9 mg sodium, 150 mg potassium, 2 g carbs, 0 g fiber, 0 sugar, 10 g protein
Serving Size	½ cup cubes
Diet Specifications	

Tomatoes

Health Benefits	Fights inflammation, supports heart health, protects bone health, stimulates digestion, balances blood pressure
Nutritional Information	1 medium whole tomato contains 22 calories, 0 fat, 0 cholesterol, 6 mg sodium, 292 mg potassium, 5 g carbs, 2 g fiber, 3 g sugar, 1 g protein
Serving Size	1 medium whole tomato
Diet Specifications	

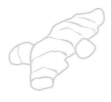

Turmeric

Health Benefits	Reduces inflammation, relieves arthritis, improves digestion, boosts liver function, lowers cholesterol
Nutritional Information	1 teaspoon contains 8 calories, 0 fat, 0 cholesterol, 1 mg sodium, 56 mg potassium, 1 g carbs, 1 g fiber, 0 sugar, 0 protein
Serving Size	1 teaspoon
Diet Specifications	

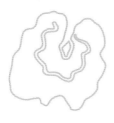

Walnuts

Health Benefits	Protects heart health, regulates blood sugar and insulin, reduces inflammation, supports bone health
Nutritional Information	1 ounce contains 185 calories, 18 g fat, 0 cholesterol, 1 mg sodium, 125 mg potassium, 4 g carbs, 2 g fiber, 1 g sugar, 4 g protein
Serving Size	1 handful
Diet Specifications	

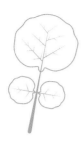

Watercress

Health Benefits	Lowers blood pressure, prevents inflammation, balances blood sugar, treats diabetes, supports bone health
Nutritional Information	1 cup contains 4 calories, 0 fat, 0 cholesterol, 14 mg sodium, 112 mg potassium, 0 carbs, 0 fiber, 0 sugar, 1 g protein
Serving Size	1 cup
Diet Specifications	

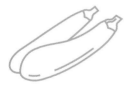

Zucchini

Health Benefits	Improves digestion, increases immunity, stabilizes blood sugar, fights infection, supports prostate health
Nutritional Information	1 medium zucchini contains 33 calories, 1 g fat, 0 cholesterol, 16 mg sodium, 512 mg potassium, 6 g carbs, 2 g fiber, 5 g sugar, 2 g protein
Serving Size	1 medium zucchini
Diet Specifications	

INDEX

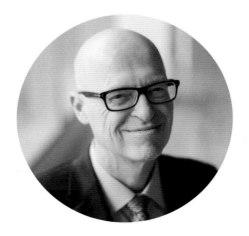

About the Author

Joshua Rosenthal is the founder, director, and primary teacher of the Institute for Integrative Nutrition®, the world's largest nutrition school, based in New York City. His innovative whole-body approach to holistic nutrition has made him a highly respected thought leader in the health and wellness space. Joshua's revolutionary concepts and teaching methods allow people to quickly and successfully reach new levels of health and happiness. Joshua holds a Master of Science degree in Education, specializing in counseling, and has over 30 years of experience in the fields of whole foods, personal coaching, curriculum development, teaching, and nutritional counseling.

About Integrative Nutrition

Founded in 1992, the Institute for Integrative Nutrition (IIN) has led the field of holistic nutrition education for more than 25 years and pioneered the concept of a Health Coach as a career. The mission of IIN is to play a crucial role in improving health and happiness, and, through that process, create a ripple effect that transforms the world. Its Health Coach Training Program allows students from all over the world to earn a Health Coach certificate. Today, 100,000 students in over 150 countries have gone through their program.

A primary concept of the curriculum is "bio-individuality," which means that no one diet works for everyone. Each and every person has unique needs. As a result, IIN is the only school in the world integrating multiple different dietary theories—combining the knowledge of traditional philosophies like Ayurveda, macrobiotics, and Chinese medicine with modern concepts like the USDA food guides, the glycemic index, The Zone, the South Beach Diet, and raw foods. In total, the curriculum covers more than 100 different dietary theories and addresses fundamental concepts, issues, and ethics of eating in a modern world. In addition, the curriculum bridges the gap between nutrition and personal growth and development through a concept called *Primary Food*. Healthy relationships, regular physical activity, fulfilling careers, and a spiritual practice feed your soul and satisfy your hunger for living. When primary food is balanced, the fun, excitement, love, and passion of your daily life nourish you on a deeper level than the food you eat.

The Health Coach Training Program also features course material on coaching techniques and running a successful business. The goal of the program is not only to provide the critical knowledge necessary in order to counsel others on nutrition, but to be an effective coach and business owner as well.

The school is a place of profound learning, with guest teachers who are the world's greatest nutrition and personal development experts, including Dr. Barry Sears, Deepak Chopra, Dr. Andrew Weil, Paul Pitchford, and Geneen Roth.

The Institute for Integrative Nutrition® graduates partner with physicians, chiropractors, fitness facilities, spas, schools, restaurants, retail stores, publishers, and corporations and work in private practice. For more information about Integrative Nutrition, visit www.integrativenutrition.com.

SPREAD THE MESSAGE OF HEALTH & HAPPINESS

Start a Career as an Integrative Nutrition Health Coach

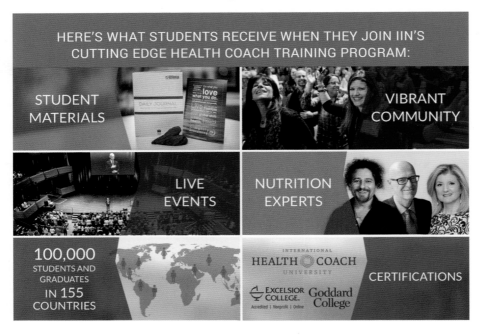

HERE'S WHAT STUDENTS RECEIVE WHEN THEY JOIN IIN'S CUTTING EDGE HEALTH COACH TRAINING PROGRAM:

STUDENT MATERIALS

VIBRANT COMMUNITY

LIVE EVENTS

NUTRITION EXPERTS

100,000 STUDENTS AND GRADUATES IN 155 COUNTRIES

CERTIFICATIONS

The Institute for Integrative Nutrition is the world's largest nutrition school and a pioneer in the field of holistic health. With 100,000 students and graduates in 155 countries, we're transforming healthcare around the world!

INTEGRATIVE NUTRITION'S ADVANCED COURSES ARE TAKING HEALTH COACHES TO THE NEXT LEVEL WITH IN-DEPTH TRAINING

- Advanced Business Course
- Launch Your Dream Book
- Coaching Mastery Course
- Hormone Health Course

- Gut Health Course
- Emotional Eating Psychology
- International Health Coach University

Visit our website to grab our curriculum guide or sign up for a free sample class!

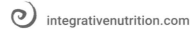

integrativenutrition.com